NCLEX-RN® Exam Medication Flashcards

Second Edition

Related Kaplan Books for Nurses

NCLEX-RN®: Strategies for the Registered Nursing Licensing Exam, 2007 Edition

Preparation for the NCLEX-RN® Exam, International Edition, Second Edition

Training Wheels for Nurses: What I Wish I Had Known My First 100 Days on the Job: Wisdom, Tips, and Warnings from Experienced Nurses

Your Career in Nursing, Third Edition

NCLEX-RN® Exam Medication Flashcards

Second Edition

Barbara Arnoldussen, R.N., M.B.A.

KAPLAN
PUBLISHING
New York • Chicago

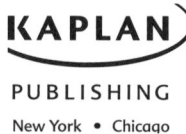

Contributing Editor: Judith A. Burckhardt
Editorial Director: Jennifer Farthing
Editor: Anne Kemper
Production Artist: Jan Gladish
Cover Designer: Carly Schnur

Published by Kaplan Publishing, a division of Kaplan, Inc.
888 Seventh Ave.
New York, NY 10106

Printed in the United States of America

June 2006
10 9 8 7 6 5 4 3

ISBN 13: 978-1-4195-7792-5
ISBN 10: 1-4195-7792-1

How to Use This Book

Kaplan's fantastic *NCLEX-RN® Exam Medication Flashcards, Second Edition* is perfectly designed to help you learn important information about 282 essential medications in a quick, easy, and fun way. Simply read the medication's category, subcategory, generic and brand names, and the phonetic pronunciation of the generic name on the front of the flashcard; then flip to the back to see its side effects, usage, and other important nursing considerations.

The following categories and subcategories have been included in the book, listed in alphabetical order by category. (Note: When the book is flipped over, the categories are listed alphabetically *from back to front.*)

Allergy and Asthma Medications

* Antihistamines
* Corticosteroids

Analgesics

* Nonopioid Analgesics
* Opioid Analgesics

Anticoagulants

Anticonvulsants

Anti-Infectives

* Aminoglycosides
* Antifungals
* Antimalarials
* Antiprotozoals
* Antituberculars
* Antivirals
* Cephalosporins, First Generation
* Cephalosporins, Second Generation
* Cephalosporins, Third Generation
* Fluoroquinolones
* Glycopeptides
* Lincosamides
* Macrolides
* Penicillins
* Sulfanamides
* Tetracyclines

Anti-Inflammatory Medications

* Corticosteroids
* Nonsteroidal Anti-Inflammatories

Antineoplastics

* Alkylating Agents
* Antimetabolites
* Hormonal Agents

Cardiovascular Medications

* ACE Inhibitors
* Alpha Blockers
* Anti-Anginals
* Anti-Arrhythmics
* Anti-Hypertensives
* Antilipemic Agents
* Beta Blockers
* Calcium Channel Blockers
* Digitalis Glycosides
* Loop Diuretics
* Platelet Aggregation Inhibitors
* Potassium-Sparing / Combination Diuretics
* Thiazides / Related Diuretics

Dermatologicals

* Antifungals, Topical
* Anti-Inflammatories, Topical

Diabetic Medications

* Hypoglycemic Agents, Oral
* Insulin
* Reversal of Hypoglycemia

Gastrointestinal Medications

* Antacids
* Anticholinergics
* Antidiarrheals
* Antiemetics
* Antiflatulents
* Anti-Ulcer Medications
* Appetite Suppressants
* Laxatives
* Pancreatic Enzymes

Genitourinary Medications

* Anticholinergics
* Anti-Impotence
* Testosterone Inhibitors
* Urinary Analgesics
* Urinary Anti-Infectives

Hormones / Synthetic Substitutes / Modifiers

* Bone Resorption Inhibitors
* Parathyroid Agents (Calcium Regulators)
* Thyroid Hormones

Mental Health Medications

* Anti-Anxiety Agents
* Antidepressants, Tricyclic
* Antidepressants, SSRIs
* Antidepressants, Other
* Antipsychotics
* Bipolar Agents

Musculoskeletal Medications
* Antigout Agents
* Nonsalicylate NSAIDs, Antirheumatics
* Salicylates, Antirheumatics
* Skeletal Muscle Relaxants

Neurological Medications

Opthalmics
* Antiglaucoma Medications
* Beta Blockers, Topical
* Opthalmics, Other

Otic (Ear) Medications

Respiratory Medications
* Antiasthmas, Other
* Antitussives
* Bronchodilators, Anticholinergic
* Bronchodilators, Sympathomimetic
* Expectorants
* Nasals, Topical

Treatment/ Replacement

* Alcohol Deterrents
* Minerals
* Narcotic Antagonists
* Vitamins

Women's Health

* Contraceptives, Systemic
* Estrogens
* Progestins

Once you've mastered a particular medication, clip or fold back the corner of the flashcard so that you can zip right by it on your next pass through the book. This flashcard book is packed with information—remember to flip the book over and flip through the other half!

Looking for still more NCLEX-RN® exam prep? Be sure to pick up a copy of Kaplan's *NCLEX-RN®: Strategies for the Registered Nursing Licensing Exam*, complete with two practice tests including 360 exam-style questions.

Good luck, and happy flipping!

Disclaimer

The material in this book is intended for study and test preparation purposes only. This book is under no circumstances to be used to prescribe medication, provide medical treatment and/or therapy, or treat patients or any other individuals in any way. The publisher is not responsible for use of this book in any manner other than its intended purpose as a study guide.

ANTIHISTAMINES

FEXOFENADINE

(fex-oh-fi-na-deen)

(Allegra)

Side Effects

Nausea

Testicular atrophy

Impotence

Contact lens intolerance

Nursing considerations

Management of abnormal uterine bleeding, secondary amenorrhea, endometrial cancer, renal cancer, contraceptive, prevent endometrial changes associated with estrogen replacement therapy

Contact clinician if weekly weight gain is over five pounds

Give IM injection deeply in large muscle mass, rotate sites, injection may be painful

Use with caution with history of depression

Contact clinician if swelling in calves, sudden chest pain or shortness of breath

(Rx; Preg Cat D)

Side Effects
Drowsiness

Nursing Considerations
Management of rhinitis, allergy symptoms, chronic idiopathic urticaria
Avoid alcohol, other CNS depressants
60 mg tablet: onset within 1 hour, peak 2–3 hours, duration about 12 hours
180 mg tablet: duration 24 hours
Rx; Preg Cat C

Women's Health

PROGESTINS

MEDROXYPROGESTRONE ACETATE

(me-drox-ee-proe-jess-te-rone)

(Provera, Depo-Provera)

HYDROXYZINE

(hye-<u>drox</u>-i-zeen)

(Atarax, Vistaril)

Side Effects

Nausea
Gynecomastia
Testicular atrophy
Impotence
Contact lens intolerance

Nursing considerations

Treatment of symptoms of menopause, inoperable breast cancer, prostatic cancer, abnormal uterine bleeding, prevention of osteoporosis

Contact clinician if breast lumps, vaginal bleeding, edema, jaundice, dark urine, clay-colored stools, dyspnea, headache, blurred vision, abdominal pain, numbness or stiffness in legs, chest pain, tenderness with redness and swelling in extremities
Men should contact clinician to report impotence or gynecomastia
Contact clinician if weekly weight gain is over five pounds
Give IM injection deeply in large muscle mass
PO: Can take with food or milk to decrease GI upset
Rx: Preg Cat X

Side Effects

Drowsiness, dry mouth

Nursing Considerations

Treatment of pruritus, pre-op anxiety, post-op nausea and vomiting, to potentiate opioid analgesics, sedation

PO: onset 15–30 minutes, duration 4–6 hours

Avoid use with alcohol, other CNS depressant

Teach pt. dizziness/drowsiness may occur; use caution in potentially hazardous activities

Rx; Preg Cat C

Women's Health

ESTROGENS

ESTROGENS CONJUGATED

(ēss-troh-genz)

(Premarin)

Allergy and Asthma Medications

ANTIHISTAMINES

LORATADINE

(lor-a-ti-deen)

(Claritin)

Side Effects

Contact lens intolerance
Gynecomastia
Testicular atrophy
Impotence

Nursing considerations

Treatment of symptoms of menopause, inoperable breast cancer (selected cases), prostatic cancer, atrophic vaginitis, prevention of osteoporosis

Contact clinician if breast lumps, vaginal bleeding, edema, jaundice, dark urine, clay-colored stools, dyspnea, headache, blurred vision, abdominal pain, numbness or stiffness in legs, chest pain, tenderness with redness and swelling in extremities

Men should contact clinician to report impotence or gynecomastia

Contact clinician if weekly weight gain is over five pounds

Apply patch to trunk of body twice a week; press firmly and hold in place for 10 seconds to ensure good contact

Rx; Preg Cat X

Side Effects

Drowsiness

Nursing Considerations

Management of seasonal rhinitis
Avoid alcohol, other CNS depressants
Take on empty stomach 1 hour before or 2 hours after meals
Onset 1–3 hours, peak 8–12 hours, duration greater than or equal to 24 hours
Rx/OTC; Preg Cat B

Women's Health

ESTROGENS

ESTRADIOL PATCH

(es-tra-dye-ole)

(Alora, Climara, Esclim, Estraderm, Fempatch)

BECLOMETHASONE

(be-kloe-meth-a-sone)

(Beclovent, Beconase)

Side Effects

Contact lens intolerance
Gynecomastia
Testicular atrophy
Impotence

Nursing considerations

Treatment of symptoms of menopause, inoperable breast cancer (selected cases), prostatic cancer, atrophic vaginitis, prevention of osteoporosis

Contact clinician if breast lumps, vaginal bleeding, edema, jaundice, dark urine, clay-colored stools, dyspnea, headache, blurred vision, abdominal pain, numbness or stiffness in legs, chest pain, tenderness with redness and swelling in extremities

Men should contact clinician to report impotence or gynecomastia

Contact clinician if weekly weight gain is over five pounds

Give IM injection deeply in large muscle mass

Rx; Preg Cat X

Side Effects

Dystonia, hoarseness
Oropharyngeal fungal infections
Headache
Sore throat
Dyspepsia

Nursing Considerations

Used in chronic asthma treatment, seasonal or perennial rhinitis
Nasal spray: onset 5–7 days, (up to 3 weeks in some patients), peak up to 3 weeks
Inhaler: onset 10 minutes
Use regular peak flow monitoring to determine respiratory status
Rx; Preg Cat C

Women's Health

ESTROGENS

ESTRADIOL CYPIONATE, ESTRADIOL VALERATE

(es-tra-dye-ole)

(Depogen, Estrasyn, Delestrogen, Valergen)

CORTICOSTEROIDS

FLUNISOLIDE

(floo-niss-oh-lide)

(Nasolide, Aerobid)

Side Effects

- Nausea
- Gynecomastia
- Testicular atrophy
- Impotence
- Contact lens intolerance

Nursing considerations

- Treatment of symptoms of menopause, inoperable breast cancer (selected cases), prostatic cancer, atrophic vaginitis, prevention of osteoporosis

Contact clinician if breast lumps, vaginal bleeding, edema, jaundice, dark urine, clay-colored stools, dyspnea, headache, blurred vision, abdominal pain, numbness or stiffness in legs, chest pain, tenderness with redness and swelling in extremities

Men should contact clinician to report impotence or gynecomastia

Contact clinician if weekly weight gain is over five pounds

Can take with food or milk to decrease GI upset

Rx; Preg Cat X

Side Effects

Dysphonia, hoarseness
Oropharyngeal fungal infections
Headache
Sore throat
Nasal congestion, cold symptoms
Nausea, vomiting, diarrhea
Unpleasant taste, upset stomach

Nursing Considerations

Used in chronic asthma treatment, seasonal or perennial rhinitis
Onset: few days
Use regular peak flow monitoring to determine respiratory status
Rx; Preg Cat C

Women's Health

ESTROGENS

ESTRADIOL (ORAL)

(es-tra-dye-ole)

(Estrace)

CORTICOSTEROIDS

FLUTICASONE

(floo-ti-ka-sone)

(Fluonase)

Side Effects

Nausea

Nursing considerations

Female contraception

Contact clinician if breast lumps, vaginal bleeding, edema, jaundice, dark urine, clay-colored stools, dyspnea, headache, blurred vision, abdominal pain, numbness or stiffness in legs, chest pain, tenderness with redness and swelling in extremities

Contact clinician if weekly weight gain is over five pounds

Can take with food or milk to decrease GI upset

Rx: Preg Cat X

Side Effects

Dysphonia, hoarseness
Oropharyngeal fungal infections
Headache
Sore throat
Nasal congestion, cold symptoms
Nausea, vomiting, diarrhea
Unpleasant taste, upset stomach

Nursing Considerations

Used in chronic asthma treatment, seasonal or perennial rhinitis
Nasal spray onset within 2 days, peak 1–2 weeks
Use regular peak flow monitoring to determine respiratory status
Rx; Preg Cat C

Women's Health

CONTRACEPTIVES, SYSTEMIC

NORGESTREL

(nor-jess-trel)

(Ovrette)

CORTICOSTEROIDS

MOMETASONE

(moe-met-a-sone)

(Nasonex)

Side Effects

Nausea

Nursing considerations

Management of abnormal uterine bleeding, amenorrhea, endometriosis, contraception

Contact clinician if breast lumps, vaginal bleeding, edema, jaundice, dark urine, clay-colored stools, dyspnea, headache, blurred vision, abdominal pain, numbness or stiffness in legs, chest pain, tenderness with redness and swelling in extremities

Contact clinician if weekly weight gain is over five pounds

Can take with food or milk to decrease GI upset

Rx; Preg Cat X

Side Effects

- Dysphonia, hoarseness
- Oropharyngeal fungal infections
- Headache
- Sore throat
- Nasal congestion, cold symptoms
- Nausea, vomiting, diarrhea
- Unpleasant taste, upset stomach

Nursing Considerations

- Used in chronic asthma treatment, seasonal or perennial rhinitis
- Nasal spray: onset few days, peak up to 3 weeks
- Use regular peak flow monitoring to determine respiratory status
- Rx; Preg Cat C

Women's Health

CONTRACEPTIVES, SYSTEMIC

NORETHINDRONE

(nor-eth-īn-drone)

(Micronor, Nor-Qd)

CORTICOSTEROIDS

TRIAMCINOLONE

(trye-am-sin-oh-lone)

(Nasocort spray, Amcort)

Side Effects

Headache

Dizziness

Nausea

Breakthrough bleeding, spotting

Nursing considerations

Prevention of pregnancy, treatment of endometriosis, hypermenorrhea (monophasic)

Contact clinician if unusual bleeding, severe headache, difficult breathing, changes in vision/coordination, chest/leg pain

Avoid smoking which increases risk of adverse cardiovascular events

Stop med for at least one week before surgery to decrease risk of thromboembolism

Rx; Preg Cat X

Side Effects

Dysphonia, hoarseness
Oropharyngeal fungal infections
Headache
Sore throat
Nasal congestion, cold symptoms
Nausea, vomiting, diarrhea
Unpleasant taste, upset stomach

Nursing Considerations

Used in chronic asthma treatment, seasonal or perennial rhinitis
Nasal spray: onset few days, peak 3–4 days
PO/IM: peak 1–2 hours
Use regular peak flow monitoring to determine respiratory status
Rx; Preg Cat C

Women's Health

CONTRACEPTIVES, SYSTEMIC

MESTRANOL/NORETHINDRONE

(mes-tre-nole nor-eth-in-drone)

(Genora, Norinyl, Ortho-Novum)

Analgesics

NONOPIOID ANALGESICS

ACETAMINOPHEN

(a-seat-a-mee-noe-fen)

(Tylenol)

Side Effects

Breakthrough bleeding

Nursing considerations

Prevention of pregnancy for 5 years as a contraceptive implant; emergency contraceptive in oral form

Implant: onset 1 month, peak 1 month, duration 5 years

Implant: six capsules are implanted in the upper arm during the first 7 days after onset of menses

PO for emergency contraceptive: Given within 72 hours of unprotected intercourse and repeated 12 hours later

Rx; Preg Cat X

Side Effects

Anemia (long-term use)
Liver and kidney failure (high prolonged doses)

Nursing Considerations

Treatment of mild pain or fever
PO: onset less than one hour, peak 1/2–2 hours, duration 4–6 hours
Rectal: onset slow, peak 1–2 hours, duration 3–4 hours
Take crushed or whole with full glass of water
Can give with food or milk to decrease GI upset
Signs of chronic poisoning: rapid, weak pulse, dyspnea, cold, clammy extremities
Signs of chronic overdose: bleeding, bruising, malaise, fever, sore throat
OTC; Preg Cat B

Women's Health

CONTRACEPTIVES, SYSTEMIC

LEVONORGESTREL

(lee-voe-nor-jess-trel)

(Norplant, Mirena)

NONOPIOID ANALGESICS

ASPIRIN

(as-pir-in)

Side Effects

Headache
Dizziness
Nausea
Breakthrough bleeding, spotting

Nursing considerations

Prevention of pregnancy, treatment of endometriosis, hypermenorrhea (monophasic)

Contact clinician if unusual bleeding, severe headache, difficulty breathing, changes in vision/coordination, chest/leg pain

Avoid smoking which increases risk of adverse cardiovascular events

Stop med for at least one week before surgery to decrease risk of thromboembolism

Rx; Preg Cat X

Side Effects

Nausea, vomiting
Rash

Nursing Considerations

Management of mild to moderate pain or fever, transient ischemic attacks, prophylaxis of MI, ischemic stroke, angina
PO: onset 15–30 minutes, peak 1–2 hours, duration 4–6 hours
Rectal: onset slow, 20–60% absorbed if retained 2–4 hours
With long-term use, check for liver damage: dark urine, clay-colored stools, yellowing of skin and sclera, itching, abdominal pain, fever, diarrhea
For arthritis, give 30 minutes before exercise; may take 2 weeks before full effect is felt
Discard tablets if vinegar-like smell
Do not give to children or teens with flulike symptoms or chickenpox; Reye's syndrome may develop
OTC; Preg Cat C

Women's Health

CONTRACEPTIVES, SYSTEMIC

ETHINYL ESTRADIOL/NORGESTREL

(eth-in-il es-tra-dye-ole nor-jess-trel)

(Ogestril, Ovral)

NONOPIOID ANALGESICS

CELECOXIB

(sel-eh-cox-ib)

(Celebrex)

Side Effects

Nausea

Nursing considerations

Female contraception (triphasic)

Contact clinician if breast lumps, vaginal bleeding, edema, jaundice, dark urine, clay-colored stools, dyspnea, headache, blurred vision, abdominal pain, numbness or stiffness in legs, chest pain, tenderness with redness and swelling in extremities

Contact clinician if weekly weight gain is over five pounds

Can take with food or milk to decrease GI upset

Rx; Preg Cat X

Side Effects

Fatigue
Anxiety, depression, nervousness
Nausea, vomiting, anorexia, dry mouth, constipation

Nursing Considerations

Management of acute, chronic arthritis pain and primary dysmenorrhea pain relief within 60 minutes
Onset: 24–48 hours, duration 12–24 hours
Can take without regard to meals
Increasing doses do not appear to increase effectiveness
Do not take if allergic to sulfonamides, aspirin, or NSAISs
Rx; Preg Cat C for first and second trimester; Preg Cat D for third trimester

Women's Health

CONTRACEPTIVES, SYSTEMIC

ETHINYL ESTRADIOL/NORETHINDRONE

(eth-in-il es-tra-dye-ole nor-eth-in-drone)

(Ortho-Novum 7-7-7)

NONOPIOID ANALGESICS

IBUPROFEN

(eye-byoo-proe-fen)

(Motrin, Advil)

Side Effects

Headache
Dizziness
Nausea
Breakthrough bleeding, spotting

Nursing considerations

Prevention of pregnancy, treatment of endometriosis, hypermenorrhea (monophasic)

Contact clinician if unusual bleeding, severe headache, difficulty breathing, changes in vision/coordination, chest/leg pain
Avoid smoking which increases risk of adverse cardiovascular events
Stop med for at least one week before surgery to decrease risk of thromboembolism
Rx; Preg Cat X

Side Effects

- Headache
- Nausea, anorexia
- GI bleeding
- Blood dyscrasias

Nursing Considerations

- Treatment of rheumatoid arthritis, osteoarthritis, primary dysmenorrhea, gout, dental pain, musculoskeletal disorders, fever
- Onset: 1/2 hour, peak 1–2 hours
- Contact clinician if ringing or roaring in ears, which may indicate toxicity
- Contact clinician if changes in urinary pattern, increased weight, edema, increased pain in joints, fever, blood in urine, which may indicate kidney damage
- Use sunscreen to prevent photosensitivity
- Avoid use with ASA, NSAIDs, and alcohol, which may precipitate GI bleeding
- OTC, Rx; Preg Cat B

Women's Health

CONTRACEPTIVES, SYSTEMIC

ETHINYL ESTRADIOL/NORETHINDRONE

(eth-in-il es-tra-dye-ole nor-eth-in-drone)

(Ortho Novum 1/35)

Analgesics

NONOPIOID ANALGESICS

NAPROXEN

(na-prox-en)

(Naprosyn, Anaprox)

Side Effects

Headache

Dizziness

Nausea

Breakthrough bleeding, spotting

Nursing considerations

Prevention of pregnancy, treatment of endometriosis, hypermenorrhea (monophasic)

Contact clinician if unusual bleeding, severe headache, difficulty breathing, changes in vision/coordination, chest/leg pain

Avoid smoking which increases risk of adverse cardiovascular events

Stop med for at least one week before surgery to decrease risk of thromboembolism

Rx; Preg Cat X

Side Effects

GI bleeding

Blood dyscrasias

Nursing Considerations

Management of mild to moderate pain. Treatment of rheumatoid, juvenile, and gouty arthritis, osteoarthritis, primary dysmenorrhea

Patients with asthma, ASA hypersensitivity or nasal polyps have increased risk of hypersensitivity

Contact clinician if blurred vision, ringing or roaring in ears, which may indicate toxicity

Contact clinician if black stools, flulike symptoms

Contact clinician if changes in urinary pattern, increased weight, edema, increased pain in joints, fever, blood in urine, which may indicate kidney damage

Avoid use with ASA, steroids and alcohol

OTC, Rx; Preg Cat B

Women's Health

CONTRACEPTIVES, SYSTEMIC

ETHINYL ESTRADIOL/ETHYNODIOL

(eth-in-il es-tra-dye-ole e-thye-noe-dye-ole)

(Demulen)

ROFOCOXIB

(roh-fih-kox-ib)

(Vioxx)

Side Effects

Headache
Dizziness
Nausea
Breakthrough bleeding, spotting

Nursing considerations

Prevention of pregnancy, treatment of endometriosis, hypermenorrhea (monophasic)
Contact clinician if unusual bleeding, severe headache, difficulty breathing, changes in vision/coordination, chest/leg pain
Avoid smoking which increases risk of adverse cardiovascular events
Stop med for at least one week before surgery to decrease risk of thromboembolism
Rx; Preg Cat X

Side Effects

Fatigue
Anxiety, depression, nervousness
Nausea, vomiting, anorexia
Dry mouth, constipation

Nursing Considerations

Management of acute, chronic arthritis pain and primary dysmenorrhea
Onset: within 45 minutes, peak 2–3 hours, duration up to 24 hours
Rx; Preg Cat C

Women's Health

CONTRACEPTIVES, SYSTEMIC

DESOGESTREL/ETHINYL ESTRADIOL

(dess-oh-jes-trel eth-in-il es-tra-dye-ole)

(Cyclessa, Desogen, Mircette, Ortho-Cept)

CODEINE

(koe-deen)

Side Effects

Headache
Nausea
Postural hypotension

Nursing Considerations

Prophylaxis and treatment of pellagra
Take with meals to reduce GI upset, can add 325 mg ASA 1/2 hour before dose to reduce flushing
Flushing will occur several hours after med taken, will decrease over 2 weeks
Avoid changing positions (sitting/standing/lying) rapidly
Rx/OTC; Preg Cat C

Side Effects

Drowsiness, sedation
Nausea, vomiting, anorexia
Respiratory depression
Constipation
Orthostatic hypotension

Nursing Considerations

Treatment of moderate to severe pain, nonproductive cough
PO: onset 30–45 minutes, peak 60–120 minutes, duration 4–6 hours
IM/subQ: onset 10–30 minutes, peak 30–60 minutes, duration 4–6 hours
Do not give if respirations are less than 12 per minute
Avoid use with alcohol, other CNS depressants
Withdrawal symptoms may occur: nausea, vomiting, cramps, fever, faintness, anorexia
Physical dependency may result from long-term use
Rx C-II, III, IV, V (depends on route); Preg Cat C

Treatment/Replacement

VITAMINS

NIACINAMIDE

(nye-ah-sīn-ah-myd)

OPIOID ANALGESICS

HYDROMORPHONE

(hye-droe-mor-fone)

(Dilaudid)

Side Effects

Diarrhea

Nursing Considerations

Treatment of Vitamin B_{12} deficiency, pernicious anemia, hemorrhage, renal and hepatic disease
IM, subQ: peak 3–10 days
Foods high in this vitamin: meats, seafood, egg yolk, fermented cheeses
OTC, Rx; Preg Cat A

Side Effects

Drowsiness, sedation
Nausea, vomiting, anorexia
Respiratory depression
Constipation, cramps
Orthostatic hypotension
Confusion, headache
Rash

Nursing Considerations

Treatment of moderate to severe pain, nonproductive cough
PO: onset 15–30 minutes, peak 30–60 minutes, duration 4–6 hours
IM: onset 15 minutes, peak 30–60 minutes, duration 4–5 hours
IV: onset 10–15 minutes, peak 15–30 minutes, duration 2–3 hours
SubQ: onset 15 minutes, peak 30–90 minutes, duration 4 hours
Rectal: duration: 6–8 hours
Do not give if respirations are less than 12 per minute
Avoid use with alcohol, other CNS depressants
Withdrawal symptoms may occur: nausea, vomiting, cramps, fever, faintness, anorexia
Physical dependency may result from long-term use
Rx C-II; Preg Cat C

Treatment/Replacement

VITAMINS

HYDROXOCOBALAMIN

(hye-drox-o-ko-bal-a-min)

(Vibral, Vitamin B_{12})

Analgesics

OPIOID ANALGESICS

MEPERIDINE

(me-per-i-deen)

(Demerol)

Side Effects

Bronchospasm

Nursing Considerations

Treatment of anemia, liver disease, alcoholism, intestinal obstruction, pregnancy

Also contained in bran, yeast, dried beans, nuts, fruits, fresh vegetables, asparagus

OTC; Preg Cat A

Side Effects

Drowsiness, sedation
Respiratory depression
Euphoria
Orthostatic hypotension
Confusion, headache

Nursing Considerations

Management of moderate to severe pain, pre-op sedation, post-op and OB analgesia
PO: onset 10–15 minutes, peak 30–60 minutes, duration 2–4 hours (usually 3)
IM: onset 10–15 minutes, peak 30–50 minutes, duration 2–4 hours (usually 3)
IV: onset less than 5 minutes, peak 5–7 minutes, duration 2–4 hours (usually 3)
SubQ: onset 10–15 minutes, peak 30–50 minutes, duration 2–4 hours (usually 3)
Do not give if respirations are less than 12 per minute
Avoid use with alcohol, other CNS depressants
Withdrawal symptoms may occur: nausea, vomiting, cramps, fever, faintness, anorexia
Physical dependency may result from long-term use
Rx C: II; Preg Cat C

Treatment/Replacement

VITAMINS

FOLIC ACID

(foe-lik a-cid)

OPIOID ANALGESICS

METHADONE

(meth-a-doan)

Side Effects

Diarrhea

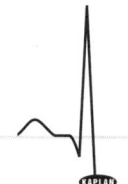

Nursing Considerations

Treatment of Vitamin B_{12} deficiency, pernicious anemia, hemorrhage, renal and hepatic disease

IM, subQ, nasal: peak 3–10 days

Foods high in this vitamin: meats, seafood, egg yolk, fermented cheeses

Excessive intake of alcohol or vitamin C may decrease oral absorption/effectiveness

OTC, Rx; Preg Cat A

Side Effects

Drowsiness, sedation
Nausea, vomiting, anorexia
Respiratory depression
Constipation, cramps
Orthostatic hypotension
Confusion, headache
Rash

Nursing Considerations

Relief of pain, detoxification/maintenance of narcotic addiction
PO: onset 30–60 minutes, peak 30–60 minutes, duration 4–6 hours (with continuous dosing, duration of action may increase to 22 to 48 hours)
IM: onset 10–20 minutes, peak 60–120 minutes, duration 4–5 hours (with continuous dosing, duration of action may increase to 22 to 48 hours)
IV: onset peak 15–30 minutes, duration 3–4 hours
Do not give if respirations are less than 12 per minute
Avoid use with alcohol, other CNS depressants
Withdrawal symptoms may occur: nausea, vomiting, cramps, fever, faintness, anorexia
Physical dependency may result from long-term use
Rx C-II; Preg Cat C

Treatment/Replacement

VITAMINS

CYANOCOBALAMIN

(sye-an-oh-koe-bal-a-min)

(Cobex, Crystamine, Cyomin)

OPIOID ANALGESICS

MORPHINE

(mor-feen)

Side Effects

Metallic taste, dry mouth

Nursing Considerations

Treatment of Vitamin D deficiency, rickets, psoriasis, rheumatoid arthritis

If med missed, omit

Decrease use of antacids and laxatives containing magnesium

Rx; Preg Cat C

Side Effects

Respiratory depression
Sedation
Euphoria
Orthostatic hypotension

Nursing Considerations

Management of severe pain
Continuous dosing is more effective than prn; may be given by patient controlled analgesia (PCA)
PO: onset 15–60 minutes, peak 30–60 minutes, duration 3–6 hours
IM: onset 10–15 minutes, peak 30–50 minutes, duration 2–4 hours (usually 3)
IV: onset less than 5 minutes, peak 18 minutes, duration 3–6 hours
SubQ: onset 10–15 minutes, peak 30–50 minutes, duration 2–4 hours (usually 3)
Withdrawal symptoms may occur: nausea, vomiting, cramps, fever, faintness, anorexia
Physical dependency may result from long-term use
Rx C-II; Preg Cat C

Treatment/Replacement

VITAMINS

CHOLECALCIFEROL (VITAMIN D_3)
ERGOCALCIFEROL (VITAMIN D_2)

(kole-e-kal-sif-e-role, er-goe-kal-sif-e-role)

(Calderol, Calciferol)

OXYCODONE

(ox-i-koe-done)

(Oxy Contin; with aspirin Percodan, with acetaminophen Percoset)

Side Effects

Withdrawal symptoms in narcotic-dependent patients: restlessness, muscle spasms, tearing

Nursing Considerations

Used to reverse narcotic depression, including respiratory symptoms

IM and subQ onset in 2 to 5 minutes; IV 1 to 2 minutes

Have emergency support equipment available

Rx; Preg Cat B

Side Effects

Drowsiness, sedation
Nausea, vomiting, anorexia
Respiratory depression
Constipation, cramps
Orthostatic hypotension
Confusion, headache
Rash
Euphoria

Nursing Considerations

Management of moderate to severe pain
PO: peak 30–60 minutes, duration 4–6 hours
Controlled release: peak 3–4 minutes, duration 12 hours
Do not give if respirations are less than 12 per minute
Avoid use with alcohol, other CNS depressants
Withdrawal symptoms may occur: nausea, vomiting, cramps, fever, faintness, anorexia
Physical dependency may result from long-term use
Rx C-II; Preg Cat B

Treatment/Replacement

NARCOTIC ANTAGONISTS

NALOXONE HCL

(nal-ox-own)

(Narcan)

PROPOXYPHENE

(proe-pox-i-feen)

(Darvon)

Side Effects

Nausea, vomiting

Cramps, diarrhea

Nursing Considerations

Prevention and treatment of hypocalemia

Onset for PO 30 minutes, IV immediate

Do not give IM, subQ

Avoid OTC antacids, salt substitutes, analgesics, vitamins unless directed

Report hyperkalemia: lethargy, confusion, GI symptoms, fainting, decreased output

Report continued hypocalemia: fatigue, weakness, polyuria, polydipsia, cardiac changes

OTC, Rx; Preg Cat C

Side Effects

Drowsiness, sedation
Nausea, vomiting, anorexia
Respiratory depression
Constipation, cramps
Orthostatic hypotension
Confusion, headache
Rash

Nursing Considerations

Management of mild to moderate pain
PO: onset 30–60 minutes, peak 120 minutes, duration 4–6 hours
Low schedule rating for misuse potential, addiction liability
Do not use in patients with suicidal tendencies
Avoid use with alcohol, other CNS depressants
Withdrawal symptoms may occur: nausea, vomiting, cramps, fever, faintness, anorexia
Physical dependency may result from long-term use with high doses
Rx C-IV; Preg Cat C

Treatment/Replacement

MINERALS

POTASSIUM

(K-Lor)

Side Effects

Nausea, constipation
Epigastric pain
Black and red tarry stools

Nursing Considerations

Treatment of iron deficiency anemia, prophylaxis for iron deficiency in pregnancy
Keep upright for 15–30 minutes to avoid esophageal corrosion, take 1 hour before bedtime
Stools will become black or dark green
Take on empty stomach, not with antacids or milk
Do not substitute one iron salt for another, since iron content differs
Rx; Preg Cat B

Anticoagulants

ANTICOAGULANTS

HEPARIN

(hep-a-rin)

Side Effects

Can produce hemorrhage from any body site (10%)
Tissue irritation/pain at injection site
Anemia
Thrombocytopenia
Fever

Nursing Considerations

Prophylaxis and treatment of thromboembolic disorders. In very low doses (10-100 units) to maintain patency of IV catheters (heparin flush)

Therapeutic PPT @ 1.5–2.5 times the control without signs of hemorrhage
IV: peak 5 minutes, duration 2–6 hours
Injection: give deep SubQ; never IM (danger of hematoma), onset 20–60 minutes, duration 8–12 hours
Antidote: protamine sulfate within 30 minutes
Signs of hemorrhage: bleeding gums, nosebleed, unusual bleeding, black, tarry stools, hematuria, fall in hematocrit or blood pressure, guaiac-positive stools
Avoid ASA-containing products and NSAIDs
Wear medical information tag
Rx; Preg Cat C

Treatment/Replacement

MINERALS

IRON POLYSACCHARIDE

(Niferex)

ANTICOAGULANTS

WARFARIN

(war-far-in)

(Coumadin)

Side Effects

Nausea, constipation

Epigastric pain

Black and red tarry stools

Nursing Considerations

Treatment of iron deficiency anemia, prophylaxis for iron deficiency in pregnancy

Contains 30% elemental iron

Keep upright for 15–30 minutes to avoid esophageal corrosion, take 1 hour before bedtime

Stools will become black or dark green

Take on empty stomach, not with antacids or milk

Do not substitute one iron salt for another, since iron content differs

Rx: Preg Cat B

Side Effects

Hemorrhage
Diarrhea
Rash
Fever

Nursing Considerations

Management of pulmonary emboli, deep-vein thrombosis, MI, atrial dysrhythmias, postcardiac valve replacement
Therapeutic PT @ 1.5–2.5 times the control, INR @ 2.0–3.0
Onset: 12–24 hours, peak 1 1/2 to 3 days; duration: 3 to 5 days
Antidote: vitamin K, whole blood, plasma
Avoid foods high in Vitamin K: many green leafy vegetables
Do not interchange brands; potencies may not be equivalent
Avoid ASA-containing products and NSAIDs
Wear medical information tag
Rx; Preg Cat X

Treatment/Replacement

MINERALS

FERROUS SULFATE

(Feosol)

ANTICONVULSANTS

CARBAMAZEPINE

(kar-ba-maz-e-peen)

(Tegretol)

Side Effects

Nausea, constipation

Epigastric pain

Black and red tarry stools

Nursing Considerations

Treatment of iron deficiency anemia, prophylaxis for iron deficiency in pregnancy

Contains 12% elemental iron

Keep upright for 15–30 minutes to avoid esophageal corrosion, take 1 hour before bedtime

Stools will become black or dark green

Take on empty stomach, not with antacids or milk

Do not substitute one iron salt for another, since iron content differs

Rx; Preg Cat B

Side Effects

Myelosuppression
Dizziness, drowsiness
Ataxia
Diplopia, rash
Photosensitivity

Nursing Considerations

Management of seizures, trigeminal neuralgia, diabetic neuropathy
Avoid driving and other activities requiring alertness the first 3 days
Monitor blood levels, CBC regularly, esp. during first 2 months; periodic eye exams
Take with food or milk to decrease GI upset; tablets (nonextended release) may be crushed, extended release capsules may be opened, mixed with juice or soft food
Urine may turn pink to brown
Avoid abrupt withdrawal; discontinue gradually
Avoid use with alcohol, other CNS depressants
Rx; Preg Cat C

Treatment/Replacement

MINERALS

FERROUS GLUCONATE

(Fergon)

Side Effects

Nausea, constipation
Epigastric pain
Black and red tarry stools

Nursing Considerations

Treatment of iron deficiency anemia, prophylaxis for iron deficiency in pregnancy
Contains 33% elemental iron
Keep upright for 15–30 minutes to avoid esophageal corrosion, take 1 hour before bedtime
Stools will become black or dark green
Take on empty stomach, not with antacids or milk
Do not substitute one iron salt for another, since iron content differs
Rx; Preg Cat B

ANTICONVULSANTS

DIVALPROEX SODIUM

(dye-val-proe-ex)

(Depakote)

Side Effects

Sedation, drowsiness, dizziness
Mental status and behavioral changes
Nausea, vomiting, constipation, diarrhea, heartburn
Prolonged bleeding time

Nursing Considerations

Management of seizures, manic episodes assoc with bipolar disorder (delayed release only), migraine prophylaxis (delayed and extended release only)
Take with or immediately after meals to lessen GI upset
Swallow tablets or capsules whole (no crushing, chewing)
Avoid abrupt withdrawal after long-term use; discontinue gradually to prevent convulsions
Monitor blood levels, platelets, bleeding time, and liver function tests
Delayed release products: peak blood level 3–5 hours, duration 12–24 hours
Extended release products: Onset 2–4 days, peak blood level 7–14 hours, duration 24 hours
Wear medical information tag
Rx; Preg Cat D

Treatment/Replacement

MINERALS

FERROUS FUMARATE

(Femiron, Feostat)

Anticonvulsants

ANTICONVULSANTS

GABAPENTIN

(ga-ba-pen-tin)

(Neurontin)

Side Effects

Nausea, constipation
Epigastric pain
Black and red tarry stools

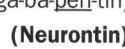

Nursing Considerations

Treatment of iron deficiency anemia in dialysis patients, given IV
Onset 4 days, peak 1–2 weeks
Stools will become black or dark green
Rx; Preg Cat C

Side Effects

- Drowsiness
- Ataxia
- Diplopia
- Rhinitis
- Constipation

Nursing Considerations

- Used for management of seizures and postherpetic neuralgia
- Do not take within 2 hours of antacid
- Avoid abrupt withdrawal after long-term use; discontinue gradually over a week to prevent convulsions
- Give without regard to meals; can open capsules and put in juice or applesauce
- Do not crush or chew capsules
- Use caution with hazardous activities
- Wear medical information tag
- Rx; Preg Cat C

Treatment/Replacement

MINERALS

FERRIC GLUCONATE COMPLEX

(Ferrlecit)

ANTICONVULSANTS

LAMOTRIGINE

(la-<u>moe</u>-tri-jeen)

(Lamictal)

Side Effects

Nausea, constipation

Epigastric pain

Black and red tarry stools

Nursing Considerations

Treatment of iron deficiency anemia, prophylaxis for iron deficiency in pregnancy

Contains 100% elemental iron

Keep upright for 15–30 minutes to avoid esophageal corrosion, take 1 hour before bedtime

Stools will become black or dark green

Take on empty stomach, not with antacids or milk

Do not substitute one iron salt for another, since iron content differs

Rx; Preg Cat B

Side Effects

Ataxia, dizziness
Headache
Nausea, vomiting, anorexia
Diplopia, blurred vision
Abdominal pain, dysmenorrhea

Nursing Considerations

Used for management of seizures
In pediatric patients, stop at first sign of rash; all patients should notify clinician of rashes
Take divided doses with meals or just after to decrease adverse effects
Use caution with hazardous activities until stabilized
Avoid abrupt withdrawal; stop gradually to prevent increase in frequency of seizures
Wear medical information tag
Rx; Preg Cat C

Treatment/Replacement

MINERALS

CARBONYL IRON

(Feosol)

ANTICONVULSANTS

PHENOBARBITAL

(fee-noe-bar-bi-tal)

(Luminal)

Side Effects

In the absence of alcohol: drowsiness, headache, restlessness, fatigue

In the presence of alcohol: flushing, chest pain, heart arrythmias, hypotension, seizures, throbbing in head and neck, sweating

Nursing Considerations

Used for treatment of chronic alcoholism by causing severe hypersensitivity

Onset may be delayed up to 12 hours; single dose may be effective for 1 to 2 weeks

Never give without patient's knowledge

Avoid alcohol in any form: in foods, sauces, or other meds, such as cough syrups or tonics

Avoid vinegar, paregoric, skin products, liniments or lotions containing alcohol

Wear medical information tag

Rx

Side Effects

- Drowsiness, lethargy, rash
- GI upset
- Initially constricts pupils
- Respiratory depression
- Ataxia

Nursing Considerations

- Management of epilepsy, febrile seizures in children, sedation, insomnia
- IV: slow rate—resuscitation equipment should be available
- IM: inject deep into large muscle mass to prevent tissue sloughing; can give subQ, onset 10–30 minutes
- PO: onset 20–60 minutes, peak 8–12 hours, duration 6–10 hours
- Use caution with hazardous activities until stabilized; drowsiness usually diminishes after initial weeks of therapy
- Nystagmus may indicate early toxicity
- Long-term use withdrawal symptoms: vomiting, sweating, abd./muscle cramps, tremors, and possibly convulsions
- Vitamin D supplements are indicated for long-term use
- Rx C-IV; Preg Cat D

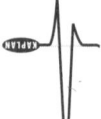

Treatment/Replacement

ALCOHOL DETERRENTS

DISULFIRAM

(dye-sul-fih-ram)

(Antabuse)

Side Effects

Nasal burning and irritation
Headache
Bad taste
Epistaxis
Postnasal drip

Nursing Considerations

Prophylaxis and treatment of allergic rhinitis
Full therapeutic effect may take several weeks
Rx; Preg Cat B

Anticonvulsants

ANTICONVULSANTS

PHENYTOIN

(fen-i-toyn)

(Dilantin)

Side Effects

- Drowsiness, ataxia
- Nystagmus
- Blurred vision
- Hirsutism
- Lethargy
- GI upset
- Gingival hypertrophy

Nursing Considerations

- Management of seizures, migraines, trigeminal neuralgia, Bell's palsy
- PO: Take divided doses, with or immediately after meals, to decrease adverse effects
- May color urine and sweat pink/red/brown
- IV administration may lead to cardiac arrest—have resuscitation equipment available; never mix in IV with any other drug or dextrose
- Avoid abrupt withdrawal to prevent convulsions
- Do not use antacids or antidiarrheals within 2 hours of med
- Use caution with hazardous activities until stabilized
- Folic acid supplements are indicated for long-term use
- Wear medical information tag
- Rx; Preg Cat C

Respiratory Medications

NASALS, TOPICAL

CROMOLYN SODIUM

(kroe-moe-lin)

(Nasalcrom)

ANTICONVULSANTS

TOPIRAMATE

(toh-pire-ah-mate)

(Topamax)

Side Effects

Nausea

Nursing Considerations

Treatment of dry, nonproductive cough

PO: onset 30 minutes, duration 4–6 hours

PO extended release: duration 12 hours

OTC, Rx, Preg Cat C

Side Effects

- Dizziness, drowsiness, fatigue
- Impaired concentration/memory
- Nervousness, speech problems
- Nausea, weight loss
- Vision problems
- Ataxia
- Photosensitivity

Nursing Considerations

- Used for management of seizures
- Give without regard to meals; can open capsules and put in juice or applesauce
- Avoid abrupt withdrawal after long-term use; discontinue gradually to prevent seizures and status epilepticus
- Use caution with hazardous activities until stabilized
- Increase fluid intake to prevent formation of kidney stones
- Stop drug immediately if eye problems; could lead to permanent loss of vision
- Use sunscreen and protective clothing to prevent photosensitivity
- Wear medical information tag
- Rx; Preg Cat C

EXPECTORANTS

GUAIFENESIN

(gwye-fen-e-sin)

(Robitussin, Mytussin)

ANTICONVULSANTS

VALPROATE

(val-proe-ate)

(Depacon)

Side Effects

Nervousness
Restlessness
Tremor

Nursing Considerations

Management of asthma or COPD
Inhalation and subQ used for short-term control; PO as long-term
PO: take with food to decrease GI upset
Tablets may be crushed and mixed with food or fluids
SubQ: Give injections in lateral deltoid
Contact clinician if unrelieved shortness of breath
Rx; Preg Cat B

Side Effects

Sedation, drowsiness, dizziness
Mental status and behavioral changes
Nausea, vomiting, constipation, diarrhea, heartburn
Prolonged bleeding time

Nursing Considerations

Used for management of seizures
Avoid abrupt withdrawal after long-term use; discontinue gradually to prevent convulsions
Monitor blood levels, platelets, bleeding time, and liver function tests
Onset of anticonvulsant effect: 2–4 days, peak blood level at end of infusion, duration 6–24 hours
Rx; Preg Cat D

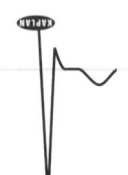

Respiratory Medications

BRONCHODILATORS, SYMPATHOMIMETIC

TERBUTALINE SULFATE

(ter-byoo-ta-leen)

(Brethine, Bricanyl)

Anticonvulsants

ANTICONVULSANTS

VALPROIC ACID

(val-proe-ic)

(Depakene, Myproic acid)

Side Effects

Headache

Nursing Considerations

Long-term control of asthma, prevention of exercise-induced asthma, prevention of bronchospasm in COPD

Do not use to treat acute symptoms; use a rapid-acting bronchodilator

Contact clinician if difficulty breathing, if more inhalations are needed of rapid-acting bronchodilator or using more than 4 inhalations of a rapid-acting bronchodilator for 2 or more consecutive days or more than 1 canister in 8 weeks

Rx; Preg Cat C

Side Effects

Sedation, drowsiness, dizziness
Mental status and behavioral changes
Nausea, vomiting, constipation, diarrhea, heartburn
Prolonged bleeding time

Nursing Considerations

Used for management of seizures
Take with or immediately after meals to lessen GI upset
Swallow capsules whole (no crushing, chewing)
Avoid abrupt withdrawal after long-term use; discontinue gradually to prevent convulsions
Monitor blood levels, platelets, bleeding time, and liver function tests
Onset: 2–4 days, peak blood level of syrup 15–120 minutes, of capsules 1–4 hours, duration 6–24 hours (varies with age)
Wear medical information tag
Rx; Preg Cat D

Respiratory Medications

BRONCHODILATORS, SYMPATHOMIMETIC

SALMETEROL

(sal-me-te-role)

(Serevent)

AMIKACIN, GENTAMICIN, TOBRAMYCIN

(am-i-kay-sin, jen-ta-mye-sin, toe-bra-mye-sin))

(Amikin, Garamycin, Tobrax)

Side Effects

Tremors
Headache
Hyperactivity
Tachycardia
Nausea, vomiting

Nursing Considerations

Treatment of bronchial asthma, reversible bronchospasm
Teach how to correctly use inhaler
Monitor for toxicity
PO: Take with food to decrease GI upset; may crush tablets
Teach how to take radial pulse
Rx; Preg Cat C–B

Side Effects

Use during pregnancy can result in bilateral congenital deafness
Ototoxicity cranial nerve VIII
Nephrotoxicity
Allergic reaction: fever, difficulty breathing, rash

Nursing Considerations

Treatment of severe systemic infections of CNS, respiratory, GI, urinary tract, bone, skin, soft tissues, acute PID
IV over 1/2 to 1 hr; IM by deep, slow injection, never subQ
Careful monitoring of blood levels
Check peak—2 hours after med given
Check trough—at time of dose/prior to med
Monitor for signs of superinfection (diarrhea, URI, coated tongue)
Immediately report hearing or balance problems
Encourage fluids to 8–10 glasses/day
Rx; Preg Cat C

Respiratory Medications

BRONCHODILATORS, SYMPATHOMIMETIC

ALBUTEROL SULFATE

(al-byoo-tear-ol)

(Proventil, Ventolin)

Anti-Infectives

ANTIFUNGALS

AMPHOTERICIN B

(am-foe-ter-i-sin)

(Fungizone)

Side Effects

Nervousness

Tremors

Dry mouth

Palpitations

Nursing Considerations

Treatment of bronchospasm assoc. with COPD, rhinorrhea, rhinitis

Not for acute bronchospasm needing rapid response

Teach use of metered dose inhaler: inhale, hold breath, exhale slowly

Don't mix in nebulizer with cromolyn sodium

Assess for hypersensitivity, including soy products, atropine, peanuts

Encourage 10–12 glasses H_2O/day

Avoid OTC cough/hayfever medications

Use caution with hazardous activities

Rx; Preg Cat B

Side Effects

Blood, kidney, heart, liver abnormalities
GI upset
Hypokalemia-induced muscle pain
CNS disturbances, inefficient hearing
Skin irritation and thrombosis if IV infiltrates

Nursing Considerations

Treatment of histoplasmosis, skin infections, septicemia, meningitis in HIV patients
Monitor vital signs; report fever or change in function, especially nervous system
Check for hypokalemia
Meticulous care and observation of injection site
Potential benefits must be balanced against serious side effects
Rx; Preg Cat B

BRONCHODILATORS, ANTICHOLINERGIC

IPRATROPIUM BROMIDE

(eye-pra-troe-pee-um)

(Atrovent)

HYDROZYCHLOROQUINE

(hye-drox-ee-klor-oh-kwin)

(Plaquenil)

Side Effects

Nausea, vomiting
Anorexia
Constipation
Circulatory and respiratory depression
Drowsiness

Nursing Considerations

Treatment of hyperactive and nonproductive cough, mild pain relief
Physical dependency may result when used for extended periods
Withdrawal symptoms may occur: nausea, vomiting, cramps, fever, faintness, anorexia
Avoid other CNS depressants
Onset: 10–20 minutes, duration 4–6 hours
Rx; Preg Cat C

Side Effects

Eye disturbances
Nausea, vomiting
Anorexia

Nursing Considerations

Management of malaria, lupus erythematosus, rheumatoid arthritis
Peak 1–2 hours
Take at the same time each day to maintain blood level
For malaria, prophylaxis should be started 2 weeks before exposure and continue for 4 to 6 weeks after leaving exposure area
Rx; Preg Cat C

ANTITUSSIVES

HYDROCODONE

(hye-droe-koe-done)

(Hycodan, with acetaminophen Vicodin)

QUININE SULFATE

(kwye-nine)

Side Effects

Dizziness

Drowsiness

Nursing Considerations

Treatment of nonproductive cough

PO: onset 15–20 minutes, duration 3–8 hours

Capsules should be swallowed whole; do not chew, because release of med may cause local anesthetic effect and choking

Additive CNS depression may occur with antihistamines, alcohol, opioids, and sedative/hypnotics

Avoid activities requiring alertness until response to med is known

Contact clinician if signs of overdose: convulsions, trembling, restlessness

Rx; Preg Cat C

Side Effects

Eye disturbances
Nausea, vomiting
Anorexia

Nursing Considerations

Treatment of malaria, nocturnal leg cramps
Peak 1–3 hours
Take at the same time each day to maintain blood level
Avoid OTC cold meds, tonic water
OTC, Rx; Preg Cat X

Respiratory Medications

ANTITUSSIVES

BENZONATE

(ben-zoe-na-tate)

(Tessalon)

ANTIPROTOZOALS

METRONIDAZOLE

(me-troe-ni-da-zole)

(Flagyl)

Side Effects

Restlessness
Dizziness
Palpitations, sinus tachycardia
Anorexia

Nursing Considerations

Treatment of bronchial asthma, bronchospasm of COPD, chronic bronchitis, emphysema
PO: peak 2 hours; take with full glass of water; best on empty stomach
Solution: peak 1 hour
Check all OTC and other meds for ephedrine before taking with this med
Avoid alcohol, caffeine, smoking
Avoid activities requiring alertness until response to med is known
Contact clinician if toxicity: nausea, vomiting, anxiety, insomnia, convulsions
Drink 8 to 10 glasses of fluid per day
Do not crush enteric-coated SR preparations, swallow whole
Rx; Preg Cat C

Side Effects
- Headache
- Dizziness
- Nausea, vomiting, diarrhea
- Abdominal cramps
- Metallic taste

Nursing Considerations
- Treatment of a wide variety of infections, including trichomoniasis and giardiasis
- IV: immediate onset, PO: peak 1–2 hours
- Urine may turn dark-reddish brown
- Avoid hazardous activities
- Treatment of both partners is necessary in trichomoniasis
- Do not drink alcohol or preparations containing alcohol during and 48 hours after use, disulfiram-like reaction can occur
- Rx; Preg Cat B

Respiratory Medications

ANTIASTHMAS, OTHER

THEOPHYLLINE

(thee-off-i-lin)

(Theo-Dur, Theovent)

Side Effects

Dizziness

Headache

Nursing Considerations

Prophylaxis and treatment of chronic asthma

Do not use to treat acute symptoms; use a rapid-acting bronchodilator

Notify clinician of wheezing, respiratory distress

Full therapeutic effect may take several weeks

Rx; Preg Cat B

ANTITUBERCULARS

ISONIAZID

(eye-soe-nye-a-zid)

(INH)

Side Effects

Peripheral neuropathy
Liver damage

Nursing Considerations

Prevention and treatment of TB
PO/IM: onset rapid, peak 1–2 hours, duration up to 24 hours
Contact clinician if signs of hepatitis: yellow eyes and skin, nausea, vomiting, anorexia, dark urine, unusual tiredness, or weakness
Contact clinician if signs of peripheral neuropathy: numbness, tingling, or weakness
Rx; Preg Cat C

Respiratory Medications

ANTIASTHMAS, OTHER

MONTELUKAST

(mon-tea-lew-cast)

(Singulair)

Anti-Infectives

ANTIVIRALS

ACYCLOVIR

(ay-sye-kloe-ver)

(Zovirax)

Side Effects

Bronchospasm
Cough
Dizziness

Nursing Considerations

Treatment of asthma
Notify clinician of wheezing, respiratory distress
Do not use for acute asthma attacks
Full therapeutic effect may take several weeks
Rx; Preg Cat B

Side Effects
Headache
Blood dyscrasias

Nursing Considerations
Treatment of herpes, varicella
IV: onset immediate, peak immediate
PO: absorbed minimally, onset unknown, peak 1 and 1/2 hours
Do not break, crush, or chew capsules
PO: Take without regard to meals with a full glass of water
If dose is missed, take as soon as remembered, up to 1 hour before next dose
Contact clinician if sore throat, fever and fatigue, could be signs of superinfection
Rx; Preg Cat B

Respiratory Medications

ANTIASTHMAS, OTHER

CROMOLYN SODIUM INHALER

(kroe-moe-lin)

(Intal)

Anti-Infectives

ANTIVIRALS

ZIDOVUDINE

(zye-doe-vue-deen)

(AZT, Retrovir)

Side Effects

Nervousness, hyperactivity
Tremors
Dry mouth, photophobia, constipation
Tachycardia, palpitations
Nausea, vomiting
Headache

Nursing Considerations

Treatment of asthma
Teach how to correctly use inhaler
Monitor for toxicity
Assess for hypersensitivity, including soy products, atropine, peanuts
Encourage 10–12 glasses H_2O/day
Avoid OTC cough/hayfever medications
Use caution with hazardous activities
Rx; Preg Cat C–B

Side Effects

Fever, headache, malaise
Dizziness
Insomnia
Dyspepsia
Nausea, vomiting, diarrhea
Anorexia
Rash

Nursing Considerations

Management of HIV infections and prevention of HIV following needlestick
GI upset and insomnia resolve after 3–4 weeks
PO: peak 1/2–1 1/2 hours
Rx; Preg Cat C

ANTIASTHMAS, OTHER

ALBUTEROL/IPRATROPIUM INHALER

(al-byoo-tear-ol/eye-pra-troe-pee-um)

(Combivent)

Anti-Infectives

CEPHALOSPORINS, FIRST GENERATION

CEFADROXIL

(sef-a-drox-ill)

(Duricef)

Nursing Considerations

Optic analgesic and antibiotic

Warn patient not to touch ear with dropper

Explain drug is for use only in ears

Rx; Preg Cat NA

Side Effects

Diarrhea

Nursing Considerations

Treatment of upper and lower respiratory tract, urinary tract, and skin infections, otitis media, tonsillitis and UTIs

Peak 1–1 1/2 hours, duration 12–24 hours

Take for 10–14 days to prevent superinfection

Rx; Preg Cat B

Optic Medications

OPTIC MEDICATIONS

HYDROCORTISONE/NEOMYCIN/POLYMIXIN OPTIC

(Cortisporin)

Nursing Considerations

Optic analgesic

Suspension: shake well (also comes in solution)

Can warm up with hands for patient's comfort

Warn patient not to touch ear with dropper

Warn patient that drug is for use only in ears

Rx; Preg Cat NA

KAPLAN

Anti-Infectives

CEPHALOSPORINS, FIRST GENERATION

CEFAZOLIN

(sef-a-zoe-lin)

(Ancef, Kefzol)

Side Effects

Diarrhea

Nursing Considerations

Treatment of upper and lower respiratory tract, urinary tract, and skin infections, bone, joint, biliary, genital infections, endocarditis, surgical prophylaxis, septicemia

IM: peak 1/2–2 hours, duration 6–12 hours

IV: peak 10 minutes, duration 6–12 hours

Rx; Preg Cat B

OPTIC MEDICATIONS

ANTIPYRINE/BENZOCAINE/GLYCERIN OPTIC SOLUTION

(Auralgan)

CEPHALOSPORINS, FIRST GENERATION

CEPHALEXIN

(sef-a-lex-in)

(Keflex)

Side Effects

Ocular irritation

Nursing Considerations

Inhibition of intraoperative miosis

Give every half hour, starting 2 hours before surgery, 4 drops to each eye

Rx; Preg Cat C

Side Effects

Diarrhea

Nursing Considerations

Treatment of upper and lower respiratory tract, urinary tract, and skin infections, bone infections, otitis media

Peak 1 hour, duration usually 6 hours, but may be up to 12 hours with decreased renal function

Take for 10–14 days to prevent superinfection

Rx; Preg Cat B

Opthalmics

OPTHALMICS, OTHER

FLURBIPROFEN

(flur-bi-proe-fen)

(Ocufen)

Anti-Infectives

CEPHALOSPORINS, FIRST GENERATION

CEPHAPIRIN

(sef-a-pye-rin)

(Cefadyl)

Side Effects

Ocular irritation

Nursing Considerations

Used in treatment of conjunctivitis, keratitis

Wash hands before and after instillation

Do not touch tip of dropper to eye or body

Do not wear soft contact lens while using this med

Rx; Preg Cat B

Side Effects

Diarrhea

Nursing Considerations

Treatment of lower respiratory tract, skin infections, endocarditis, bacterial peritonitis

IM: peak 30 minutes, duration 4–6 hours

IV: peak 5 minutes, duration 4–6 hours

Rx; Preg Cat B

Opthalmics

OPTHALMICS, OTHER

CROMOLYN NA

(kroe-moe-lin)

(Opticrom)

CEPHALOSPORINS, FIRST GENERATION

CEPHRADINE

(<u>sef</u>-ra-deen)

(Velosef)

Side Effects

Ocular hyperemia
Allergic conjunctivitis
Pruritus

Nursing Considerations

Treatment of glaucoma and ocular hypertension
Wait 15 minutes after use to wear soft contact lens
Use caution with hazardous activities due to decreased mental alertness
Avoid alcohol
Monitor intraocular pressure because may reverse after 1 month of therapy
Rx; Preg Cat B

Side Effects

Diarrhea

Nursing Considerations

Treatment of serious respiratory tract and skin infections, otitis media, and UTIs

Peak 1–2 hours, duration usually 6 hours, but may be up to 12 hours with decreased renal function

Take for 10–14 days to prevent superinfection

Rx; Preg Cat B

Opthalmics

OPTHALMICS, OTHER

BRIMONIDINE TARTRATE

(brih-moh-nih-deen)

(Alphagan)

Anti-Infectives

CEPHALOSPORINS, SECOND GENERATION

CEFACLOR

(sef-a-klor)

(Ceclor)

Side Effects

Fatigue
Weakness

Nursing Considerations

Treatment of glaucoma and ocular hypertension
Place pressure on tear ducts for one minute
Wash hands before and after instillation
Do not touch drug container to eye or body
Rx; Preg Cat C

Side Effects

Diarrhea

Nursing Considerations

Treatment of respiratory tract, urinary tract, bone, joint and skin infections, otitis media

Peak 1/2–1 hour, extended release peak 1 1/2–2 1/2 hours

Take for 10–14 days to prevent superinfection

Rx; Preg Cat B

Opthalmics

BETA BLOCKERS, TOPICAL

TIMOLOL

(tim-oh-lole)

(Timoptic gel, Betimol solution)

Side Effects

Hypotension

Transient eye stinging and burning

Asthma attacks in patients with history of asthma

Nursing Considerations

Treatment of glaucoma and ocular hypertension

Place pressure on tear ducts for one minute

Wash hands before and after instillation

Do not touch tip of dropper to eye or body

Drug is a beta blocker.

Although given topically, it can be absorbed systemically

Report shortness of breath, chest pain or heart irregularity

Wear medical identification tag

Rx; Preg Cat C

CEPHALOSPORINS, SECOND GENERATION

CEFAMANDOLE

(sef-a-man-dole)

(Mandol)

Side Effects

Diarrhea

Nursing Considerations

Treatment of respiratory tract, urinary tract, and skin infections, peritonitis, septicemia, surgical prophylaxis
Peak 1/2–1 hour
IV or IM
Avoid alcohol
Rx; Preg Cat B

Opthalmics

BETA BLOCKERS, TOPICAL

LEVOBUNOLOL

(lee-voe-byoo-no-lole)

(AK-beta, Betagan)

CEPHALOSPORINS, SECOND GENERATION

CEFDITOREN PIVOXIL

(sef-dit-oh-ren pih-vox-il)

(Spectracef)

Side Effects

Ocular hyperemia
Decreased visual acuity
Eye discomfort or pain
Foreign body sensation
Eye pruritus

Nursing Considerations

Treatment of glaucoma and ocular hypertension for patient who can't tolerate or responds inadequately to other IOP-lowering drugs
Place pressure on tear ducts for one minute
Wash hands before and after instillation
Do not touch tip of dropper to eye or body
Potential for increased brown pigmentation of iris, eyelid skin darkening, changes in eyelashes, important if only one eye being treated
Stop if eye inflammation or eyelid reactions
Remove contact lens to give med, can reinsert in 15 minutes
Discard med six months after opening
Rx; Preg Cat C

Side Effects

Diarrhea

Nursing Considerations

Treatment of acute bacterial exacerbation of chronic bronchitis, pharyngitis/tonsilitis, uncomplicated skin infections

Peak 1 1/2–3 hours

Take for 10–14 days to prevent superinfection

Rx; Preg Cat B

Opthalmics

ANTIGLAUCOMA MEDICATIONS

TRAVOPROST

(trav-oh-prahst)

(Travatan)

CEPHALOSPORINS, SECOND GENERATION

CEFONICID

(se-fon-i-sid)

(Monocid)

Side Effects

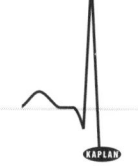

Ocular burning, stinging, discomfort
Blurred vision, tearing, or dryness
Photophobia
Bitter taste in mouth

Nursing Considerations

Treatment of glaucoma and ocular hypertension
Place pressure on tear ducts for one minute
Wash hands before and after instillation
Do not touch drug container to eye or body
Do not wear contact lens during instillation
Drug contains sulfonamide. Although given topically, it can be absorbed systemically
Stop if eye inflammation or eyelid reactions
Rx; Preg Cat C

Side Effects
Diarrhea

Nursing Considerations
Treatment of respiratory tract, urinary tract, skin infections, otitis media, peritonitis, septicemia
IM: peak 1 hour
IV: onset 5 minutes
Rx; Preg Cat B

Opthalmics

ANTIGLAUCOMA MEDICATIONS

DORZOLAMIDE/TIMOLOL

(dor-zoh-la-mide tye-moe-lole)

(Cosopt)

Side Effects

Ocular burning, stinging, discomfort
Blurred vision, tearing, or dryness
Photophobia
Bitter taste in mouth

Nursing Considerations

Treatment of glaucoma and ocular hypertension
Wash hands before and after instillation
Do not touch tip of dropper to eye or body
Do not wear contact lens during instillation
Drug is a sulfonamide. Although given topically, it can be absorbed systemically
Stop if eye inflammation or eyelid reactions
Rx; Preg Cat C

Anti-Infectives

CEPHALOSPORINS, SECOND GENERATION

CEFOTETAN

(sef-oh-tee-tan)

(Cefotan)

Side Effects

Diarrhea

Nursing Considerations

Treatment of respiratory tract, urinary tract, bone, joint and skin infections, GYN and gonococcal infections, intrabdominal infections

IM/IV: peak 1 1/2–3 hours or at end of infusion

Avoid alcohol

Rx; Preg Cat B

Opthalmics

ANTIGLAUCOMA MEDICATIONS

DORZOLAMIDE HCL

(dor-zoh-la-mide)

(Trusopt)

CEPHALOSPORINS, SECOND GENERATION

CEFOXITIN

(se-fox-i-tin)

(Mefoxin)

Side Effects

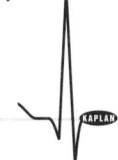

Weakness, neck stiffness

Tingling, hot sensation, burning, feeling of pressure, tightness

Numbness, dizziness, sedation

Nursing Considerations

Used for treatment of acute migraine with or without aura

Take with fluids as soon as symptoms occur

PO: Tablet may be split

Avoid foods high in tyramine: cheese, pickled products, alcohol, large amounts of caffeine

Rx; Preg Cat C

Side Effects

Diarrhea

Nursing Considerations

Treatment of respiratory tract, urinary tract, bone and skin infections, GYN and gonococcal infections, peritonitis, septicemia
IM: peak 20–30 minutes
IV: peak at end of infusion
Take for 10–14 days to prevent superinfection
Avoid alcohol
Eat yogurt or buttermilk to maintain intestinal flora
Rx; Preg Cat B

ZOLMITRIPTAN

(zole-mih-trip-tan)

(Zomig)

CEPHALOSPORINS, SECOND GENERATION

CEFPROZIL

(sef-proe-zill)

(Cefzil)

Side Effects

Dizziness

Cardiac dysrhythmias

Nursing Considerations

Indirect acting dopaminergic agent

Used in management of Parkinson's disease with levodopa/carbidopa

Do not use with tricyclics or opioids

Monitor for signs of toxicity: twitching, eye spasms

Do not stop abruptly; parkinsonian crisis may occur

Avoid foods high in tyramine: cheese, pickled products, alcohol, large amounts of caffeine

Rx, Preg Cat C

Side Effects

Diarrhea

Nursing Considerations

Treatment of pharyngitis/tonsilitis, otitis media, secondary bacterial infection of acute bronchitis, and acute bacterial exacerbation of chronic bronchitis, acute sinusitis

Peak 1 1/2 hours

Take for 10–14 days to prevent superinfection

Rx; Preg Cat B

Neurological Medications

NEUROLOGICAL MEDICATIONS

SELEGILINE

(se-lē-ji-leen)

(Eldepryl)

CEPHALOSPORINS, SECOND GENERATION

CEFUROXIME

(sef-yoor-ox-eem)

(Ceftin)

Side Effects

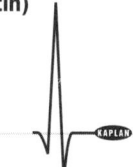

Hyperactivity, insomnia

Restlessness, talkativeness

Palpitations, tachycardia

Nursing Considerations

Management of attention deficit hyperactive disorder, narcolepsy, depression in the elderly

Onset 1/2 hour, duration 4–6 hours

Take at least 6 hours before bedtime (regular release) or 10 hours before bedtime (sustained release, extended release)

Taper med over several weeks, or depression, increased sleeping, lethargy will occur

Avoid hazardous activities until stabilized on med

Decrease caffeine consumption (coffee, tea, cola, chocolate) to decrease irritability

Rx; C-II; Preg Cat C

Side Effects

Diarrhea

Nursing Considerations

Treatment of respiratory tract, urinary tract, bone and skin infections, gonococcal infections, meningitis, septicemia

Take for 10–14 days to prevent superinfection

Rx; Preg Cat B

NEUROLOGICAL MEDICATIONS

METHYLPHENIDATE

(meth-ill-fen-i-date)

(Ritalin)

CEPHALOSPORINS, SECOND GENERATION

LORACARBEF

(lor-a-kar-beff)

(Lorabid)

Side Effects

Twitching
Headache, dizziness
Dark urine/sweat
Cardiac arrhythmias
Mental changes: confusion, agitation, mood alterations

Nursing Considerations

Replacement dopaminergic agent
Change positions slowly
Take with food, decreased effect with liver, pork, wheat germ and vitamin B6
Full therapeutic effect may take several weeks to a few months
Rx; Preg Cat NA

Side Effects
Diarrhea

Nursing Considerations
Treatment of respiratory tract, urinary and skin infections, otitis media, pharyngitis, tonsilitis
Peak 1 hour
Take for 10–14 days to prevent superinfection
Rx; Preg Cat B

NEUROLOGICAL MEDICATIONS

LEVODOPA

(leev-oe-doe-pa)

(Dopar, Larodopa)

CEPHALOSPORINS, THIRD GENERATION

CEFDINIR

(sef-dih-ner)

(Omnicef)

Side Effects

Nausea, vomiting, diarrhea
Headache
Insomnia
Seizures

Nursing Considerations

Used in treatment of mild to moderate dementia
Drug does not cure but stabilizes or relieves symptoms
Take at regular intervals
Take between meals or may be given with meals to decrease
GI upset
Rx; Preg Cat C

Side Effects

Nausea, vomiting, diarrhea
Anorexia

Nursing Considerations

Treatment of acute exacerbations of chronic bronchitis
Take for 10–14 days to prevent superinfection
Rx; Preg Cat B

Neurological Medications

NEUROLOGICAL MEDICATIONS

DONEPEZIL

(don-ep-ee-zill)

(Aricept)

CEPHALOSPORINS, THIRD GENERATION

CEFEPIME

(sef-e-peem)

(Maxipime)

Side Effects

Twitching
Headache, dizziness
Dark urine/sweat
Cardiac arrhythmias
Mental changes: confusion, agitation, mood alterations

Nursing Considerations

Replacement dopaminergic agent
Change positions slowly
Take with food, decreased effect with liver, pork, wheat germ, and vitamin B6
Full therapeutic effect may take several months
Rx; Preg Cat NA

Side Effects

Nausea, vomiting, diarrhea
Anorexia

Nursing Considerations

Treatment of respiratory tract, urinary, and skin infections
IV: peak 1/2 hour
IM: peak 2 hours
Rx; Preg Cat B

NEUROLOGICAL MEDICATIONS

CARBIDOPA/LEVODOPA

(leev-oe-doe-pa)

(Sinemet)

Side Effects

Headache
Tremors, convulsions
Blood vessel contraction, with decreased circulation, esp. limbs
Toxic ergotism: nausea, vomiting, diarrhea, dizziness, headache, mental confusion

Nursing Considerations

Treatment of vascular headache
Take at onset of pain/during prodomal stage to abort headache
Lie down in darkened quiet room for several hours
Rx; Preg Cat X

CEPHALOSPORINS, THIRD GENERATION

CEFOPERAZONE

(sef-oh-per-a-zone)

(Cefobid)

Side Effects

Nausea, vomiting, diarrhea
Anorexia

Nursing Considerations

Treatment of respiratory tract, urinary, bone and skin infections, bacterial septicemia, peritonitis, PID
anorexia
IV: onset 5 minutes, peak 5–20 minutes, duration 6–8 hours
IM: peak 1–2 hours, duration 6–8 hours
Avoid alcohol
Rx; Preg Cat B

Neurological Medications

NEUROLOGICAL MEDICATIONS

CAFFEINE/ERGOTAMINE

(er-got-a-meen)

(Cafergot)

Side Effects

Dry mouth

Constipation

Nursing Considerations

Treatment of Parkinson symptoms, EPS associated with neuroleptic drugs, acute dystonic reactions

IM/IV: onset 15 minutes, duration 6–10 hours

PO: onset 1 hour, duration 6–10 hours

Tablets may be crushed and mixed with food

Taper med over a week, or withdrawal symptoms: EPS, tremors, insomnia, tachycardia, restlessness

Avoid hazardous activities until stabilized on med

Change positions slowly

Avoid alcohol, antihistamines unless directed

Rx; Preg Cat C

CEPHALOSPORINS, THIRD GENERATION

CEFOTAXIME

(sef-oh-taks-eem)

(Claforan)

Side Effects

Nausea, vomiting, diarrhea
Anorexia

Nursing Considerations

Treatment of respiratory tract, intra-abdominal/GYN infections, gonococcal infections, meningitis, septicemia, bacteremia
IV: onset 5 minutes
IM: onset 30 minutes
Rx; Preg Cat B

BENZTROPINE

(benz-troe-peen)

(Cogentin)

CEPHALOSPORINS, THIRD GENERATION

CEFPODOXIME

(sef-poe-docks-eem)

(Vantin)

Side Effects

Drowsiness

Dizziness

Light-headedness

Nausea

Nursing Considerations

Relieves muscle spasms from acute conditions, tetanus management

IM: Inject deep into UOQ of buttock, rotate sites

NG tube: Crush tablets into fluid

PO: Take with food or milk

Metallic taste may develop

Urine may turn green, black or brown

Avoid alcohol, other CNS depressants, including OTC cold or allergy meds

Avoid activities requiring alertness until effects known

Rx; Preg Cat C

Side Effects

Nausea, vomiting, diarrhea
Anorexia

Nursing Considerations

Treatment of respiratory tract, urinary tract, and skin infections, otitis media and STD infections
Take for 10–14 days to prevent superinfection
Rx; Preg Cat B

Musculoskeletal Medications

SKELETAL MUSCLE RELAXANTS

METHOCARBAMOL

(meth-oh-kar-ba-mole)

(Robaxin)

CEPHALOSPORINS, THIRD GENERATION

CEFTAZIDIME

(sef-tay-zi-deem)

(Tazidime)

Side Effects

Drowsiness
Dizziness
Dry mouth
Constipation

Nursing Considerations

Relieves muscle spasms from acute conditions
Avoid alcohol, other CNS depressants, including OTC cold or allergy meds
Avoid activities requiring alertness until effects known
Rx; Preg Cat B

Side Effects

Nausea, vomiting, diarrhea
Anorexia

Nursing Considerations

Treatment of respiratory tract, urinary tract, GYN, joint, bone and skin infections, gonococcal infections, meningitis, septicemia, intra-abdominal infections
IV/IM: peak 1 hour or at end of infusion
Rx; Preg Cat B

Musculoskeletal Medications

SKELETAL MUSCLE RELAXANTS

CYCLOBENZAPRINE

(sye-kole-ben-za-preen)

(Flexeril)

Anti-Infectives

CEPHALOSPORINS, THIRD GENERATION

CEFTIBUTEN

(sef-ti-byoo-tin)

(Cedax)

Side Effects

Drowsiness
Dizziness
Light-headedness
Nausea

Nursing Considerations

Relief of pain, stiffness
PO: onset 1/2 hour, peak 4 hours, duration 4–6 hours
Avoid alcohol, other CNS depressants, including OTC cold or allergy meds
Avoid activities requiring alertness until effects known
Rx; Preg Cat C

Side Effects

Nausea, vomiting, diarrhea
Anorexia

Nursing Considerations

Treatment of pharyngitis and tonsilitis, otitis media, secondary bacterial infection of acute bronchitis
Peak 2–3 hours
Take for 10–14 days to prevent superinfection
Rx; Preg Cat B

Musculoskeletal Medications

SKELETAL MUSCLE RELAXANTS

CARISOPRODOL

(kar-eye-soe-proe-dole)

(Soma)

CEPHALOSPORINS, THIRD GENERATION

CEFTIZOXIME

(sef-ti-zox-eem)

(Cefizox)

Side Effects

Drowsiness

Dizziness

Weakness, fatigue

Confusion

Nausea, vomiting

Nursing Considerations

Used to reduce spasticity in multiple sclerosis, spinal cord injury

Take with food

Avoid alcohol, other CNS depressants

Increased risk of seizures in patients with seizure disorder

Withdraw gradually over 1 to 2 weeks, unless severe adverse reactions; D/C may cause hallucinations, tachycardia or rebound spasticity

Monitor for symptoms of sensitivity: fever, skin eruptions, respiratory distress

Rx; Preg Cat C

Side Effects

Nausea, vomiting, diarrhea
Anorexia

Nursing Considerations

Treatment of respiratory tract, urinary tract, bone, joint and skin infections, PID, meningitis, septicemia, intra-abdominal infections
IV: onset 5 minutes depending on length of infusion
IM: peak 1 hour
Rx; Preg Cat B

BACLOFEN

(bak-loe-fen)

SKELETAL MUSCLE RELAXANTS

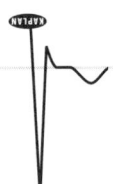

Musculoskeletal Medications

Anti-Infectives

FLUOROQUINOLONES

CIPROFLOXACIN

(sip-ro-flocks-a-sin)

(Cipro)

Side Effects

Nausea, vomiting
GI bleeding
Heartburn
Rash

Nursing Considerations

For mild to moderate pain
PO: can be crushed or whole
PO: take with food or milk to decrease GI upset
Full therapeutic effect may take 2 weeks
Read label on OTC meds, may contain ASA
Monitor for signs of toxicity: changes in liver, kidney, eye, ear functions
Rx; Preg Cat C

Side Effects

Seizures
Nausea, vomiting, diarrhea, abd. distress, flatulence
Rash
Photosensitivity

Nursing Considerations

Treatment of infection caused by E. coli and other bacteria, chronic bacterial prostatis, acute sinusitis, postexposure inhalation anthrax
Contraindicated in children less than 18 years of age
Take 2 hours pc or 2 hours before an antacid or iron preparation
Take at equal intervals around the clock
Avoid caffeine
Encourage fluids to 8–10 glasses/day
Rx; Preg Cat C

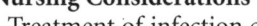

Musculoskeletal Medications

SALICYLATES, ANTIRHEUMATICS

SALSALATE

(sal-sah-late)

(Disalcid)

VANCOMYCIN

(van-koe-mye-sin)

(Lyphocin, Vancocin, Vancoled)

Side Effects

Drowsiness
Headache

Nursing Considerations

For mild to moderate pain
PO: with food to decrease GI upset; on empty stomach to increase absorption
Take at same time every day
Monitor for signs of toxicity: blurred vision, ringing or roaring in ears
Full therapeutic effect may take up to 1 month
Avoid concurrent use of ASA, other OTC meds, alcohol
Rx; Preg Cat B

Side Effects

Liver damage

Nursing Considerations

Treatment of resistant staph infections, colitis, staph enterocolitis, endocarditis prophylaxis for dental procedures (used for c. difficile)

PO: poor absorption

IV: peak 5 minutes, duration 12–24 hours

Give antihistamine if "red man syndrome": decreased blood pressure, flushing of face and neck

Contact clinician if signs of superinfection: sore throat, fever, fatigue

Rx; Preg Cat C

NONSALICYLATE NSAIDS, ANTIRHEUMATICS

PIROXICAM

(peer-ox-i-kam)

(Feldene)

Anti-Infectives

LINCOSAMIDES

CLINDAMYCIN HCL PHOSPHATE

(klin-da-my-sin)

(Cleocin HCl, Cleocin Phosphate for IM)

Side Effects

Nausea
Dizziness
Headache

Nursing Considerations

For mild to moderate pain
PO: with food to decrease GI upset; on empty stomach to increase absorption
Monitor for signs of toxicity: blurred vision, ringing or roaring in ears
Full therapeutic effect may take up to 1 month
Avoid concurrent use of ASA, steroids, alcohol
(Rx/OTC); Preg Cat B

Side Effects

Nausea, vomiting, diarrhea
Abdominal pain
Vaginitis

Nursing Considerations

Treatment of infections caused by staph, strep, and other organisms
PO: peak 45 minutes, duration 6 hours
IM: peak 3 hours, duration 8–12 hours
Rx; Preg Cat B

Musculoskeletal Medications

NONSALICYLATE NSAIDS, ANTIRHEUMATICS

NAPROXEN NA

(na-prox-en)

(Naprosyn)

Anti-Infectives

MACROLIDES

AZITHROMYCIN

(ay-zi-thro-my-sin)

(Zithromax)

Side Effects

Peptic ulcer
Dizziness
Bone marrow depression
Drowsiness
Blurred vision

Nursing Considerations

Treatment of rheumatoid arthritis/osteoarthritis, acute gout, acute painful shoulder

Observe for bleeding problems
PO: Take with food/milk, encourage upright position for 15–30 minutes
Use caution with potentially hazardous activities
Avoid use with alcohol, aspirin, other NSAIAs
Rx; Preg Cat NA

Side Effects

Nausea, vomiting, diarrhea

Nursing Considerations

Treatment of mild to moderate infections of the respiratory tract, skin, nongonoccocal urethritis, cervicitis, acute pharyngitis/tonsillitis, community acquired pneumonia

PO: rapid onset, peak 2.5–3.2 hours, duration 24 hours

IV: rapid onset, peak end of infusion, duration 24 hours

PO: don't take with antacids; can take with or without food

Monitor for signs of superinfection (diarrhea, perineal itching, oral ulcers)

If treated for nongonococcal urethritis or cervicitis, sexual partners also need treatment

Rx; Preg Cat B

Musculoskeletal Medications

NONSALICYLATE NSAIDS, ANTIRHEUMATICS

INDOMETHACIN

(in-doe-meth-a-sin)

(Indocin)

Anti-Infectives

MACROLIDES

ERYTHROMYCIN

(eh-rith-roe-<u>mye</u>-sin)

(Ery-Tab, Erythrocin)

Side Effects

Nausea, vomiting, diarrhea, constipation

Headache, dizziness

Fluid retention

Nursing Considerations

Treatment of rheumatoid arthritis/osteoarthritis; relief of mild/moderate pain; antipyretic

Take with milk or food

Use cautiously with aspirin allergy

Rx/OTC; Preg Cat NA

Side Effects

Abdominal cramps
Pain at injection site
Nausea, vomiting, diarrhea

Nursing Considerations

Treatment of infections, including chlamydia, syphilis
PO: Give 1 hr ac/2 hr pc with full glass H_2O (avoid citrus juice); some formulations can be given without regard to meals
PO: onset 1 hour, peak up to 4 hours, duration 6–12 hours
IV: onset rapid, peak end of infusion, duration 6–12 hours
Take at equal intervals around the clock
Can be used in patients with compromised renal function
Monitor for signs of superinfection (diarrhea, perineal itching, oral ulcers)
Rx; Preg Cat B

Musculoskeletal Medications

NONSALICYLATE NSAIDS, ANTIRHEUMATICS

IBUPROFEN

(eye-byoo-proe-fen)

(Advil, Motrin)

Anti-Infectives

PENICILLINS

AMOXICILLIN, AMPICILLIN, PENICILLIN

(ah-mox-ih-sill-in, am-pih-sill-in, pen-i-sill-in)

(Amoxil, Omnipen, Bicillin, Wycillin)

Side Effects

Nephrotoxicity
Nausea
Anorexia
Dizziness
Blood dyscrasias

Nursing Considerations

Reduces pain of osteoarthritis
Monitor for signs of toxicity: blurred vision, ringing or roaring in ears
Full therapeutic effect may take up to 1 month
Avoid concurrent use of ASA, NSAIDs, acetaminophen, alcohol
Rx; Preg Cat C

Side Effects

Allergic reactions: fever, difficulty breathing, skin rash
Renal, hepatic, hematologic abnormalities
Nausea, vomiting, diarrhea

Nursing Considerations

Treatment of respiratory infections, scarlet fever, otitis media, pneumonia, skin and soft tissue infections, gonorrhea
Take careful history of penicillin reaction; observe for 20 minutes post IM injection
PO for penicillin and ampicillin: Take 1 hr ac or 2 hrs pc to reduce gastric acid destruction of drug. Not true for amoxicillin
Take equally divided doses around the clock
Continue medication for entire time prescribed, even if symptoms resolve
Check for hypersensitivity to other drugs, esp. cephalosporins
Rx; Preg Cat B

NONSALICYLATE NSAIDS, ANTIRHEUMATICS

ETODOLAC

(ee-toe-doe-lak)

(Lodine)

SULFISOXAZOLE

(sul-fi-<u>sox</u>-a-zole)

(Gantrisin)

KAPLAN

Side Effects

Dizziness
Headache
Nephrotoxicity
Blood dyscrasias

Nursing Considerations

Used in arthritic conditions, dysmenorrhea
Ophthalmic: reduce inflammation after cataract extraction
PO: Take with full glass of water and food and remain upright for 1/2 hour
If dose missed, take within 2 hours
Use sunscreen to prevent photosensitivity
Rx; Preg Cat B

Side Effects

Headache
Nausea, vomiting, diarrhea
Allergic rash
Urinary crystallization
Photosensitivity

Nursing Considerations

Treatment of urinary tract, systemic infections, chancroid, trachoma, toxoplasmosis, acute otitis media, malaria (adjunctive therapy), meningitis, eye infections
PO: full glass H_2O
Monitor I and 0, force fluids
Rx; Preg Cat C

NONSALICYLATE NSAIDS, ANTIRHEUMATICS

DICLOFENAC NA

(dye-kloe-fen-ak)

(Voltaren)

TRIMETHOPRIM-SULFAMETHOXAZOLE

(trye-meth-oh-prim-sul-fa-meth-ox-a-zole)

(Bactrim, Septra)

Side Effects

Nausea
Skin rash
Hemolytic anemia
Sore gums, anorexia

Nursing Considerations

Treatment of hyperuricemia assoc. with gout, gouty arthritis
Check BUN, renal function tests
Encourage 8–10 glasses H_2O/day
Give with milk, food, and antacids
Avoid use of alcohol, eating organ meats, gravy, legumes
Avoid aspirin-containing products, may take acetaminophen

Side Effects

Hypersensitivity reaction
Blood dyscrasias
Stop at first sign of skin rash
Photosensitivity

Nursing Considerations

Treatment of urinary tract, chancroid, acute otitis media, acute and chronic prostatitis, shigellosis, pneumoonitis, chronic bronchitis, traveler's diarrhea

PO: with full glass H_2O; if upset stomach occurs, take with food
PO: Take at equal intervals around the clock
IV solution must be given slowly over 60–90 minutes; flush lines at end of infusion to remove residual
Never administer IM, rapidly IV, or by bolus injection
Encourage fluids to 8–10 glasses/day
Rx: Preg Cat C

ANTIGOUT AGENTS

PROBENECID

(proe-ben-e-sid)

(Benemid)

Anti-Infectives

TETRACYCLINES

DOXYCYCLINE HYCLATE

(dox-i-sye-kleen)

(Vibramycin)

Side Effects

Nausea, vomiting, diarrhea
Agranulocytosis
Sign of toxicity: abdominal cramps

Nursing Considerations

Treatment and prevention of acute gout attacks
Has analgesic, anti-inflammatory effects
Take with food/milk
IV: slowly; do not administer IM/subQ
Encourage 10–12 glasses H_2O/day
Avoid use of alcohol, eating organ meats, gravy, legumes
Always carry medication to treat acute attacks
Rx; Preg Cat D

Side Effects

Photosensitivity
GI upset, diarrhea
Renal, hepatic, hematologic abnormalities
Dental discoloration of deciduous (baby) teeth

Nursing Considerations

Treatment of syphilis, chlamydia, gonorrhea, malaria prophylaxis, chronic periodontitis, acne
Peak 1 1/2–4 hours
If GI symptoms occur, administer with food EXCEPT milk products or other foods high in calcium (interferes with absorption)
Take with full glass of water, do NOT take within 1 hr of bedtime or reclining
Check patient's tongue for Monilia infection
Discard outdated prescriptions
Avoid prolonged exposure to direct sunlight, UV light
Avoid during tooth and early development periods (4th month prenatal to 8 years of age)
Rx; Preg Cat D

ANTIGOUT AGENTS

COLCHICINE

(kol-chi-seen)

MINOCYCLINE HCL

(mi-noe-sye-kleen)

(Minocin)

Side Effects

GI upset

Headache, drowsiness

Rash

Nursing Considerations

Treatment of gout, uric acid neuropathy, uric acid stone formation

Encourage 10–12 glasses H_2O/day

Check CBC and renal function tests

Take with food; don't take vitamin C or iron

Initial therapy can increase attacks

Avoid use of alcohol, eating organ meats, gravy, legumes

Full therapeutic effect may require several months

Rx; Preg Cat C

Side Effects

Photosensitivity
GI upset, diarrhea
Renal, hepatic, hematologic abnormalities
Dental discoloration of deciduous (baby) teeth

Nursing Considerations

Treatment of chlamydia, periodontitis, acne
Peak 2–3 hours
If GI symptoms occur, administer with food EXCEPT milk products or other foods high in calcium (interferes with absorption)
Take with full glass of water, do NOT take within 1 hr of bedtime
Check patient's tongue for Monilia infection
Discard outdated prescriptions
Avoid prolonged exposure to direct sunlight, UV light
Avoid during tooth and early development periods (4th month prenatal to 8 years of age)
Rx; Preg Cat D

Musculoskeletal Medications

ANTIGOUT AGENTS

ALLOPURINOL

(al-oh-pure-i-nole)

(Aloprim, Zyloprim)

CORTICOSTEROIDS

DEXAMETHASONE

(dex-a-meth-a-sone)

(Decadron)

Side Effects

Dizziness
Impaired vision
Fine hand tremors
Reversible leukocytosis
Signs of intoxication: vomiting, diarrhea, drowsiness, muscular weakness, ataxia

Nursing Considerations

Controls manic episodes in manic depressive individuals; mood stabilizer
Use caution in potentially hazardous activities
Check serum levels 2 times weekly during treatment, q 2–3 mos on maintenance; draw blood in AM prior to dose
Target serum levels: treatment = .5 to 1.5 mEq/L, maintenance = .6–1.2mEq/L
GI symptoms reduced if taken with meals
Onset of therapeutic effects in 1–2 weeks
Diabetics: closely monitor blood/urine glucose
Dose reduced during depressive stages of illness
Encourage 10–12 glasses H_20/day and adequate salt intake (6–10 grams/day)
Avoid caffeine, increased exercise, saunas
Rx; Preg Cat D

Side Effects

Depression
Flushing, sweating
Hypertension
Nausea, diarrhea
Abdominal distention
Increased appetite

Nursing Considerations

Treatment of inflammation, allergies, neoplasms, collagen disorders
PO: Take with food, milk, antacids
Excessive consumption of licorice can increase risk of hypokalemia
Eat food high in potassium, protein, calcium, vitamin D; avoid sodium
Contact clinician if anorexia, difficulty breathing, weakness, dizziness
Contact clinician if black/tarry stools, slow wound healing, blurred vision, bruising/bleeding, weight gain, emotional changes
Wear medical identification tag
Rx; Preg Cat C

Mental Health Medications

BIPOLAR AGENTS

LITHIUM

(li-thee-um)

(Lithobid, Eskalith)

DEXAMETHASONE ACETATE, DEXAMETHASONE SODIUM PHOSPHATE

(dex-a-meth-a-sone)

(Decadron-LA, Decadron Phosphate)

Side Effects

Sedation, drowsiness, dizziness
Mental status and behavioral changes
Nausea, vomiting, constipation, diarrhea, heartburn
Prolonged bleeding time

Nursing Considerations

Management of seizures, manic episodes assoc. with bipolar disorder (delayed release only), migraine prophylaxis (delayed and extended release only)
Take with or immediately after meals to lessen GI upset
Swallow tablets or capsules whole (no crushing, chewing)
Avoid abrupt withdrawal after long-term use; discontinue gradually to prevent convulsions
Monitor blood levels, platelets, bleeding time, and liver function tests
Delayed release products: peak blood level 3-5 hours, duration: 12–24 hours
Extended release products: peak blood level 7–14 hours, duration: 24 hours
Wear medical information tag
Rx; Preg Cat D

Side Effects

Depression
Flushing, sweating
Hypertension
Nausea, diarrhea
Abdominal distention
Increased appetite

Nursing Considerations

Treatment of inflammation, allergies, neoplasms, cerebral edema, septic shock, collagen disorders
IV: use sodium phosphate form, not acetate (injection suspension)
IM: shake suspension well, give deep into gluteal UOQ, avoid deltoid, rotate sites
Excessive consumption of licorice can increase risk of hypokalemia
Eat food high in protein, calcium, vitamin D; avoid sodium
Contact clinician if anorexia, difficulty breathing, weakness, dizziness
Contact clinician if black/tarry stools, slow wound healing, blurred vision, bruising/bleeding, weight gain, emotional changes
Wear medical identification tag
Rx; Preg Cat C

Mental Health Medications

BIPOLAR AGENTS

DIVALPROEX SODIUM

(dye-val-proe-ex)

(Depakote)

Anti-Inflammatory Medications

CORTICOSTEROIDS

HYDROCORTISONE

(hy-dro-kor-tih-sone)

(Cortef, Solu-Cortef)

Side Effects

Myelosuppression
Dizziness, drowsiness
Ataxia
Diplopia, rash
Photosensitivity

Nursing Considerations

Management of bipolar disorder, seizures, trigeminal neuralgia, diabetic neuropathy
Avoid driving and other activities requiring alertness the first 3 days
Monitor blood levels, CBC regularly, esp. during first 2 months; periodic eye exams
Take with food or milk to decrease GI upset; tablets (non extended release) may be crushed, extended release capsules may be opened, mixed with juice or soft food
Urine may turn pink to brown
Avoid abrupt withdrawal; discontinue gradually
Avoid use with alcohol, other CNS depressants
Patient should wear medical information tag
Rx; Preg Cat C

Side Effects

Depression
Flushing, sweating
Hypertension
Nausea, diarrhea

Nursing Considerations

Treatment of severe inflammation, septic shock, adrenal insufficiency, ulcerative colitis, collagen disorders
Med masks signs of infection, so check for elevated temperature, WBC count
PO: Take with food, milk, antacids
IM: give deep into gluteal UOQ, avoid deltoid, rotate sites, avoid subQ administration since it may damage tissue
Rectal: for colitis, retain med for 20 minutes, onset 3–5 days
Wear medical identification tag
Rx; Preg Cat C

BIPOLAR AGENTS

CARBAMAZEPINE

(kar-ba-maz-e-peen)

(Tegretol)

CORTICOSTEROIDS

METHYLPREDNISOLONE

(meth-ill-pred-niss-oh-lone)

(Medrol)

Side Effects

Drowsiness
Dizziness
Tardive dyskinesia
Constipation

Nursing Considerations

Used in treatment of psychotic states
Avoid use with alcohol, other CNS depressants
Use caution in potentially hazardous activities
Avoid changing positions (lying/sitting/standing) rapidly
Notify clinician if fever, sore throat, bruising/bleeding, tics/spasms, trembling, shuffling gait
Avoid strenuous exercise in hot weather
Check before taking OTC meds
Women: avoid breast-feeding
Rx; Preg Cat C

Side Effects

Peptic ulcer/possible perforation
Hypertension and circulatory problems
Poor wound healing

Nursing Considerations

Treatment of severe inflammation, shock, adrenal insufficiency, management of acute spinal cord injury, collagen disorders
PO: Take with food, milk, antacids
PO: peak 1–2 hours, duration 1 1/2 days
IM: give deep into gluteal UOQ, avoid deltoid, rotate sites, avoid subQ administration, since it may damage tissue
IM: peak 4–8 days, duration 1–4 week
Eat food high in protein, calcium, vitamin D; avoid sodium
Contact clinician if anorexia, difficulty breathing, weakness, dizziness; symptoms may appear during periods of stress or trauma
Contact clinician if black/tarry stools, slow wound healing, blurred vision, bruising/bleeding, weight gain, emotional changes
Wear medical identification tag
Rx; Preg Cat C

Mental Health Medications

ANTIPSYCHOTICS

ZIPRASIDONE HCL

(zye-praz-i-doan)

(Geodon)

CORTICOSTEROIDS

PREDNISOLONE

(pred-niss-oh-lone)

(Prelone, Cortalone)

Side Effects

Drowsiness
Dizziness

Nursing Considerations

Used in treatment of psychotic states
Avoid use with alcohol, other CNS depressants
Use caution in potentially hazardous activities
Avoid changing positions (lying/sitting/standing) rapidly
Notify clinician if fever, sore throat, bruising/bleeding, tics/spasms, trembling, shuffling gait
Avoid strenuous exercise in hot weather
Check before taking OTC meds
Rx; Preg Cat C

Side Effects

Depression
Hypertension, circulatory problems
Nausea, diarrhea
Abdominal distention

Nursing Considerations

Treatment of severe inflammation, imunosuppression, neoplasms
PO: Take with food, milk, antacids
PO: duration 18–36 hours
IM: give deep into gluteal UOQ, avoid deltoid, rotate sites, avoid subQ administration, since it may damage tissue
IM: peak 3–45 hours
Eat food high in protein, calcium, vitamin D; avoid sodium
Contact clinician if anorexia, difficulty breathing, weakness, dizziness; symptoms may appear during periods of stress or trauma
Contact clinician if black/tarry stools, slow wound healing, blurred vision, bruising/bleeding, weight gain, emotional changes
Wear medical identification tag
Rx; Preg Cat C

Mental Health Medications

ANTIPSYCHOTICS

QUETIAPINE

(kweh-tie-a-peen)

(Seroquel)

Anti-Inflammatory Medications

CORTICOSTEROIDS

PREDNISONE

(pred-ni-sone)

(Cordrol, Deltasone, Predacort)

Side Effects

- Drowsiness
- Dizziness
- Tardive dyskinesia
- Constipation

Nursing Considerations

- Treatment of psychotic states
- Avoid use with alcohol, other CNS depressants
- Use caution in potentially hazardous activities
- Avoid changing positions (lying/sitting/standing) rapidly
- Notify clinician if fever, sore throat, bruising/bleeding, tics/spasms, trembling, shuffling gait
- Avoid strenuous exercise in hot weather
- Check before taking OTC meds
- Rx; Preg Cat C

Side Effects

Peptic ulcer/possible perforation
Depression
Hypertension, circulatory problems
Nausea, diarrhea
Abdominal distention

Nursing Considerations

Treatment of severe inflammation, immunosuppression, neoplasms, multiple sclerosis, collagen disorders, dermatologic disorders

PO: Take with food, milk, antacids
PO: peak 1–2 hours, duration 1–1/2 days
Eat food high in protein, calcium, vitamin D; avoid sodium
Contact clinician if anorexia, difficulty breathing, weakness, dizziness; symptoms may appear during periods of stress or trauma
Contact clinician if black/tarry stools, slow wound healing, blurred vision, bruising/bleeding, weight gain, emotional changes
Excessive consumption of licorice can increase risk of hypokalemia
Wear medical identification tag
Rx; Preg Cat C

ANTIPSYCHOTICS

RISPERIDONE

(riss-pair-i-doan)

(Risperdal)

NONSTEROIDAL ANTI-INFLAMMATORIES

CELECOXIB

(sel-eh-cox-ib)

(Celebrex)

Side Effects

- Drowsiness
- Dizziness

Nursing Considerations

- Treatment of psychotic states, Tourette syndrome
- PO concentrate: dilute with water, not coffee or tea
- PO: Take with food or full glass of water/milk
- IM: Inject slowly, deep into UOQ of buttock; have patient lie down for 1/2 hour
- Avoid abrupt withdrawal; discontinue gradually
- Avoid use with alcohol, other CNS depressants
- Use caution in potentially hazardous activities
- Avoid changing positions (lying/sitting/standing) rapidly
- Wear protective clothing, sunglasses due to photosensitivity
- Rx; Preg Cat C

Side Effects

Fatigue
Anxiety, depression, nervousness
Nausea, vomiting, anorexia
Dry mouth, constipation

Nursing Considerations

Treatment of rheumatoid arthritis, osteoarthritis, primary dysmenorrhea, acute pain
Peak 3 hours
Take without regard to food, but with a full glass of water to enhance absorption
Avoid use with other NSAIDs, aspirin, which can have cross hypersensitivity with sulfonamides
Blacks show a 40 percent increase in total amount absorbed compared with Caucasians
Take at about the same time daily
Rx; Preg Cat C for first and second trimester; Preg Cat D for third trimester

Mental Health Medications

ANTIPSYCHOTICS

HALOPERIDOL

(ha-loe-per-i-dole)

(Haldol)

NONSTEROIDAL ANTI-INFLAMMATORIES

IBUPROFEN

(eye-byoo-proe-fen)

(Motrin, Advil)

Side Effects

Abnormal dreams, insomnia
Anxiety, nervousness
Dizziness, weakness
Headache
Abdominal pain
Nausea, vomiting, diarrhea
Anorexia, weight loss
Sexual dysfunction
Sedation

Nursing Considerations

Treatment of major depression or relapse, generalized anxiety disorder
Take with food; extended release tablets should be swallowed whole
If dose missed, take immediately unless time for next dose
May require gradual reduction before stopping if taken over 6 weeks
Avoid use with alcohol, other CNS depressants for up to one week after end of therapy
Use caution in potentially hazardous activities
Avoid changing positions (lying, sitting, standing) rapidly
Rx: Preg Cat C

Side Effects

Headache
Nausea, anorexia
GI bleeding
Blood dyscrasias

Nursing Considerations

Treatment of rheumatoid arthritis, osteoarthritis, primary dysmenorrhea, gout, dental pain, musculoskeletal disorders, fever
Onset: 1/2 hour, peak 1–2 hours,
Contact clinician if blurred vision, ringing or roaring in ears, which may indicate toxicity
Contact clinician if changes in urinary pattern, increased weight, edema, increased pain in joints, fever, blood in urine, which may indicate kidney damage
Full therapeutic effect may take up to 1 month
Avoid use with ASA, NSAIDs, and alcohol, which may precipitate GI bleeding
OTC, Rx; Preg Cat B

Mental Health Medications

ANTIDEPRESSANTS, OTHER

VENLAFAXINE

(ven-lah-fax-een)

(Effexor)

NONSTEROIDAL ANTI-INFLAMMATORIES

NAPROXEN

(na-prox-en)

(Naprosyn, Anaprox)

Side Effects

Drowsiness
Hypotension
Dry mouth
Nausea
Dizziness
Priapism

Nursing Considerations

Treatment of major depression
Take with or immediately after meals to lessen GI upset
If dose missed, take it immediately, unless within 4 hours of next dose
May require gradual reduction before stop
Avoid use with alcohol, other CNS depressants for up to one week after end of therapy
Use caution in potentially hazardous activities
Avoid changing positions (lying, sitting, standing) rapidly
Rx; Preg Cat C

Side Effects

GI bleeding
Blood dyscrasias

Nursing Considerations

Management of mild to moderate pain. Treatment of rheumatoid, juvenile, and gouty arthritis, osteoarthritis, primary dysmenorrhea

Patients with asthma, ASA hypersensitivity, or nasal polyps have increased risk of hypersensitivity

Contact clinician if blurred vision, ringing or roaring in ears, which may indicate toxicity

Contact clinician if black stools, flulike symptoms

Contact clinician if changes in urinary pattern, increased weight, edema, increased pain in joints, fever, blood in urine, which may indicate kidney damage

Use sunscreen to prevent photosensitivity

Avoid use with ASA, steroids and alcohol

OTC, Rx; Preg Cat B

Mental Health Medications

ANTIDEPRESSANTS, OTHER

TRAZODONE

(tray-zoe-doan)

(Desyrel)

NONSTEROIDAL ANTI-INFLAMMATORIES

ROFOCOXIB

(roh-fih-kox-ib)

(Vioxx)

Side Effects

Drowsiness, dizziness
Constipation
Dry mouth
Increased appetite, weight gain

Nursing Considerations

Treatment of depression
Do not use within 14 days of MAO inhibitor
May require gradual reduction before stopping
Check with clinician before taking OTC cold remedy
Avoid use with alcohol, other CNS depressants for up to one week after end of therapy
Use caution in potentially hazardous activities
Rx; Preg Cat C

Side Effects

Fatigue
Anxiety, depression, nervousness
Nausea, vomiting, anorexia
Dry mouth, constipation

Nursing Considerations

Management of acute, chronic arthritis pain and primary dysmenorrhea
Onset: within 45 minutes, peak 2–3 hours, duration up to 24 hours
Take without regard to food, but with a full glass of water to enhance absorption
Avoid other NSAIDs, aspirin, alcohol
Patients with asthma, aspirin allergy, or nasal polyps may be hypersensitive
Rx; Preg Cat C

ANTIDEPRESSANTS, OTHER

MIRTAZAPINE

(mer-taz-e-peen)

(Remeron)

ANTINEOPLASTICS

METHOTREXATE

(meth-oh-trex-ate)

(Trexall)

Side Effects

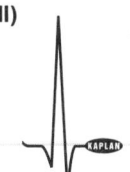

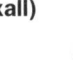

Agitation
Headache
Dry mouth
Nausea, vomiting
Tremor

Nursing Considerations

Treatment of depression and smoking cessation
If missed dose for depression, take as soon as possible and space remaining doses at not less than 4 hour intervals.
If missed dose for smoking cessation, omit dose
May require gradual reduction before stopping
Avoid use with alcohol, other CNS depressants for up to one week after end of therapy
Use caution in potentially hazardous activities
Avoid changing positions (lying, sitting, standing) rapidly
Rx; Preg Cat B

Side Effects

Nausea, vomiting, diarrhea
Anorexia
Alopecia

Nursing Considerations

Treatment of cancer, mycosis fungoides, psoriasis, rheumatoid arthritis
PO, IM, IV: onset 4–7 days, peak 7–14 days, duration 21 days
Avoid crowds or people with known infections
Do not take ASA or other NSAIDs which may cause GI bleeding
Monitor for pulmonary toxicity, which may manifest early as a dry, nonproductive cough
Rx; Preg Cat X

Mental Health Medications

ANTIDEPRESSANTS, OTHER

BUPROPION HCL

(byoo-proe-pee-on)

(Wellbutrin, Zyban)

Antineoplastics

ANTINEOPLASTICS

TAMOXIFEN

(ta-mox-i-fen)

(Nolvadex)

Side Effects

Headache
Dizziness
Tremor
Insomnia
Nausea, diarrhea
Dry mouth
Male sexual dysfunction

Nursing Considerations

Treatment of depression, OCD, panic disorder with or without agoraphobia, PTSD
Take consistently at same time of day; therapeutic effects take up to four weeks
Can potentiate effects of digoxin, Coumadin, and Valium
Used for anorexia, not suicidal or homicidal emotions
Avoid use with alcohol, other CNS depressants for up to one week after end of therapy
Use caution in potentially hazardous activities
Rx; Preg Cat B

Side Effects

Nausea, vomiting
Hot flashes
Rash

Nursing Considerations

Management of advanced breast cancer not responsive to other therapy in estrogen-receptor-positive patients
Peak 4–7 hours
To decrease GI upset, take after antacid, after evening meal, before bedtime, or take antiemetic 30–60 minutes ahead
Vaginal bleeding, pruritus, hot flashes are reversible after stopping med
Contact clinician if decreased visual acuity, which may be irreversible
Tumor flare (increase in tumor size and increased bone pain) may occur, but will decrease rapidly; may take analgesics for pain
Rx; Preg Cat D

Mental Health Medications

ANTIDEPRESSANTS, SSRI'S

SERTRALINE HCL

(sīr-trah-leen)

(Zoloft)

ACE INHIBITORS

CAPTOPRIL

(kap-toe-pril)

(Capoten)

KAPLAN

Side Effects

Palpitations
Nausea, vomiting, diarrhea, or constipation
Decreased appetite
Nervousness, insomnia

Nursing Considerations

Treatment of anxiety, depression, OCD and social anxiety disorder, panic disorder, PTSD
Take consistently at same time of day; therapeutic effects in up to four weeks
Avoid use with alcohol, other CNS depressants for up to one week after end of therapy
Use caution in potentially hazardous activities
Rx; Preg Cat C

Side Effects

Dizziness
Orthostatic hypotension
Tachycardia
Bronchospasm, dyspnea, cough
Loss of taste

Nursing Considerations

Treatment of hypertension, CHF, left ventricular dysfunction after MI, diabetic neuropathy
Contact clinician if fever, skin rash, sore throat, mouth sores, swelling of hands or feet, fast or irregular heartbeat, chest pain, or cough
Take on empty stomach 1 hour before meals or 2 hours after; tablets may be crushed and mixed with juice or soft food for ease of swallowing
Loss of taste might last for first 2–3 months, clinical concern is interference with nutrition
Avoid changing positions (sitting/standing/lying) rapidly, esp. during the first few days, before body adjusts to med
Do not use OTC (cough, cold or allergy) meds unless directed by clinician
Avoid potassium supplements and K salt substitute
Rx; Preg Cat First Trimester C; Second Trimester D

Mental Health Medications

ANTIDEPRESSANTS, SSRI'S

PAROXETINE HCL

(pair-ox-eh-teen)

(Paxil)

ACE INHIBITORS

ENALAPRIL

(e-<u>nal</u>-a-pril)

(Vasotec)

Side Effects

- Palpitations
- Nausea, diarrhea, or constipation
- Decreased appetite with significant weight loss
- Nervousness, insomnia
- Urinary retention
- Drowsiness
- Rash, pruritus, excessive sweating
- Fatigue

Nursing Considerations

- Treatment of depression/OCD, bulimia
- Take consistently at same time of day; full therapeutic effects may require four weeks
- Can potentiate effects of digoxin, Coumadin, and Valium
- Used for anorexia, not suicidal or homicidal emotions
- Avoid use with alcohol, other CNS depressants for up to one week after end of therapy
- Use caution in potentially hazardous activities
- Rx; Preg Cat B

Side Effects

- Headache
- Dizziness, hypotension
- Tachycardia
- Tinnitus
- Hyperkalemia

Nursing Considerations

- Treatment of hypertension, CHF, left ventricular dysfunction
- Contact clinician if fever, skin rash, sore throat, mouth sores, swelling of hands or feet, fast or irregular heartbeat, chest pain, or cough
- Avoid changing positions (sitting/standing/lying) rapidly, esp. during the first few days, before body adjusts to med
- Cardiovascular adverse reactions may reoccur
- Do not use OTC (cough, cold, or allergy) meds unless directed by clinician
- Avoid potassium supplements and potassium salt substitutes
- Rx; Preg Cat First Trimester C; Second Trimester D

Mental Health Medications

ANTIDEPRESSANTS, SSRI'S

FLUOXETINE HCL

(floo-ox-uh-teen)

(Prozac)

FOSINOPRIL

(foh-sin-oh-prill)

(Monopril)

Side Effects

Palpitations, bradycardia
Nausea, vomiting, diarrhea
Decreased appetite
Nervousness, insomnia
Drowsiness

Nursing Considerations

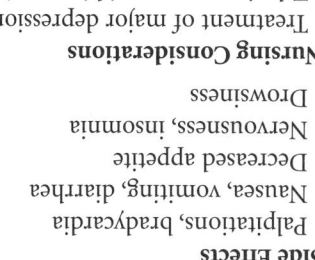

Treatment of major depression
Take in A.M. to avoid insomnia
Can potentiate effects of digoxin, Coumadin, and Valium
Avoid use with alcohol, other CNS depressants for up to one week after end of therapy
Use caution in potentially hazardous activities
Avoid changing positions (lying, sitting, standing) rapidly
Take consistently at same time of day; therapeutic effects in up to four weeks
Rx; Preg Cat C

Side Effects

Headache
Dizziness, fatigue
Nausea, vomiting, diarrhea

Nursing Considerations

Treatment of hypertension, adjunct in treating CHF when not responding to usual meds
Take at the same time each day; peaks at 2–6 hours
Initial response might include dizziness and lightheadedness
Avoid salt substitutes containing potassium
Change positions (sitting/standing/lying) slowly
Contact clinician if sore throat, swelling of hands and feet, chest pain, mouth sores, irregular heart beat
Rx; Preg Cat D

ANTIDEPRESSANTS, SSRI'S

CITALOPRAM

(sit-al̄-oh-pram)

(Celexa)

ACE INHIBITORS

LISINOPRIL

(lye-sin-oh-pril)

(Prinivil, Zestril)

Side Effects

Sedation/drowsiness
Blurred vision, dry mouth, diaphoresis
Postural hypotension, palpitations
Nausea, vomiting, diarrhea
Constipation, urinary retention
Increased appetite
Sexual dysfunction

Nursing Considerations

Treatment of major depression
Avoid use with alcohol, other CNS depressants
Suicide risk high after 10–14 days, due to increased energy
Increase fluid intake
Take dose at bedtime due to sedative effect
Heavy smokers may require a larger dose
Use safety precautions with hazardous activity
Avoid sudden positional changes, partial hypotension
Women: avoid use if pregnant, breast-feeding
Rx; Preg Cat C

Side Effects

Headache
Dizziness
Hypotension
Tachycardia
Nausea, vomiting, diarrhea
Fatigue

Nursing Considerations

Treatment of mild to moderate hypertension, systolic CHF, acute MI
Avoid changing positions (lying/sitting/standing) rapidly
May take without regard to food
Avoid high sodium foods (canned soups, lunch meats, cheese)
Avoid high potassium foods (bananas, citrus fruits, raisins)
Rx; Preg Cat First Trimester C; Second Trimester D

Mental Health Medications

ANTIDEPRESSANTS, TRICYCLIC

NORTRIPTYLINE

(nor-trip-ti-leen)

(Pamelor)

ACE INHIBITORS

RAMIPRIL

(ram-ih-prill)

(Altace)

Side Effects

Sedation/drowsiness
Dry mouth
Postural hypotension, palpitations
Diarrhea
Urinary retention
Anorexia

Nursing Considerations

Treatment of depression, enuresis in children
Full therapeutic effect may take 2–3 weeks
Drug is dispensed in small amounts at beginning of treatment due to suicide potential
Use safety precautions with hazardous activity
Avoid sudden positional changes
Do not stop abruptly: could cause nausea, malaise, headache
Avoid alcohol, other CNS depressants
Rx; Preg Cat C

Side Effects

Headache
Dizziness
Vertigo
Hypotension
Nausea

Nursing Considerations

Treatment of hypertension, CHF following MI, reduce risk of death from CV causes in patients with risk factors
Can mix capsule contents with water, juice, or applesauce to aid swallowing
Avoid changing positions (lying/sitting/standing) rapidly
Contact clinician if persistent, dry, nonproductive cough, increased SOB, edema, or unusual bruising or bleeding
Avoid salt substitutes containing potassium
Rx; Preg Cat D

Mental Health Medications

ANTIDEPRESSANTS, TRICYCLIC

IMIPRAMINE

(im-ip-ra-meen)

(Tofranil, Tipramine)

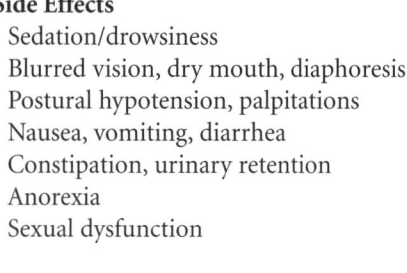

Cardiovascular Medications

ALPHA BLOCKERS

DOXAZOSIN MESYLATE

(dox-ay-zoe-sin)

(Cardura)

Side Effects

Sedation/drowsiness
Blurred vision, dry mouth, diaphoresis
Postural hypotension, palpitations
Nausea, vomiting, diarrhea
Constipation, urinary retention
Anorexia
Sexual dysfunction

Nursing Considerations

Treatment of major depression, anxiety
Avoid use with alcohol
Suicide risk high after 10–14 day due to increased energy
Increase fluid intake
Take dose at bedtime, due to sedative effect
Heavy smokers may require a larger dose
Use safety precautions with hazardous activity
Avoid sudden positional changes
Rx; Preg Cat C

Side Effects

Dizziness
Headache
Fatigue, malaise

Nursing Considerations

Treatment of hypertension, benign prostatic hyperplasia (BPH)
Avoid changing positions (lying/sitting/standing) rapidly
Can have first dose syncope, maintain recumbent for 90 minutes
Wear medical identification tag
Full therapeutic effects may require several weeks of therapy
Avoid high sodium foods (canned soups, lunch meats, cheese)
Use caution in potentially hazardous activities until stabilized
Avoid alcohol, smoking
Rx; Preg Cat B/C

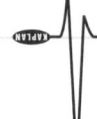

Mental Health Medications

ANTIDEPRESSANTS, TRICYCLIC

DOXEPIN

(dox-e-pin)

(Adapin, Sinequan)

ALPHA BLOCKERS

PRAZOSIN HCL

(pray-zoh-sin)

(Minipress)

Side Effects

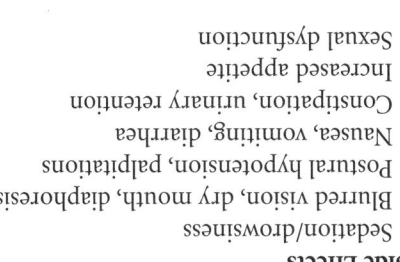

Sedation/drowsiness
Blurred vision, dry mouth, diaphoresis
Postural hypotension, palpitations
Nausea, vomiting, diarrhea
Constipation, urinary retention
Increased appetite
Sexual dysfunction

Nursing Considerations

Treatment of major depression
Suicide risk high after 10–14 days due to increased energy
Avoid use with alcohol
Sun block required
Increase fluid intake
Take dose at bedtime due to sedative effect
Heavy smokers may require a larger dose
Use safety precautions with hazardous activity
Avoid sudden positional changes, partial hypotension
Rx: Preg Cat C

Side Effects

Dizziness
Drowsiness
Headache
Nausea, vomiting, diarrhea
Palpitations

Nursing Considerations

Treatment of hypertension
Onset 2 hours, peak 1–3 hours, duration 6–12 hours
Can have first dose syncope, take the first dose (and any increment) at bedtime, do not drive for 24 hours
Full therapeutic effects may require 4 to 6 weeks of therapy
Food may delay absorption and minimize side effects
Avoid changing positions (lying/sitting/standing) rapidly
Check with clinician before using OTC cold, cough and allergy meds
Rx; Preg Cat C

ANTIDEPRESSANTS, TRICYCLIC

AMITRIPTYLINE

(a-mee-trip-ti-leen)

(Elavil)

Cardiovascular Medications

ALPHA BLOCKERS

TERAZOSIN HCL

(ter-ay-zoh-sin)

(Hytrin)

Side Effects

Dizziness, drowsiness
Orthostatic hypotension
Blurred vision

Nursing Considerations

Management of anxiety, irritability in psychiatric or organic disorders, preoperatively, insomnia, adjunct in endoscopic procedures
PO: onset 30 minutes, peak 1–6 hours
IM: Onset 15–30 minutes, peak 1–1 1/2 hours
IV: Onset 5–15 minutes, peak unknown
May be taken with food
May be habit forming; do not take for longer than 4 months unless directed
Avoid alcohol, other CNS depressants
Do not stop drug abruptly
Drowsiness may worsen at beginning of treatment
Rx; Preg Cat D

Side Effects

Dizziness
Headache
Drowsiness
Nausea

Nursing Considerations

Treatment of hypertension, benign prostatic hyperplasia (BPH)
Avoid changing positions (lying/sitting/standing) rapidly
Can have first dose syncope, take the first dose (and any increment) at bedtime, do not drive or operate machinery for 4 hours
Rx; Preg Cat C

Mental Health Medications

ANTI-ANXIETY AGENTS

LORAZEPAM

(lor-ā-ze-pam)

(Ativan)

ISOSORBIDE DINITRATE

(eye-soe-sor-bide)

(Isordil)

Side Effects

Drowsiness, fatigue, ataxia
Hypotension
Paradoxic anxiety, esp. in elderly
Orthostatic hypotension
Blurred vision

Nursing Considerations

Treatment of anxiety, acute alcohol withdrawal, seizures; pre-operative and skeletal muscle relaxant

PO: May be taken with food, onset 1/2 hour

IM: inject deep, slowly into large muscle mass; inset 15–30 minutes, duration 1–1 1/2 hours, slow and erratic absorption

IV: into large vein, push doses should not exceed 5 mg/minute, resuscitation equipment available; onset immediate, duration 15 minutes–1 hour

Smoking may decrease effectiveness

Avoid use with alcohol, other CNS depressants

Long-term use withdrawal symptoms: vomiting, sweating, abd./muscle cramps, tremors, and possibly convulsions

May be habit-forming if used over 4 months

Rx C-IV; Preg Cat NA

Side Effects

Dizziness, postural hypotension
Vascular headache, flushing
Drowsiness
Nausea

Nursing Considerations

Treatment/prophylaxis of angina pectoris, CHF
PO: 1 hour before food or 2 hours after meals for maximum absorption, but taking with food may reduce or eliminate headache
Chewable tablet: chew well, hold in mouth for 2 minutes before swallowing
Sublingual: dissolve under tongue, do not eat, drink, talk or smoke during use, go to ED if pain not relieved in 15 minutes
Avoid changing positions (lying/sitting/standing) rapidly
Use caution in potentially hazardous activities until stabilized
Avoid alcohol, smoking, strenuous exercise in hot environment
Wear medical identification tag
Rx; Preg Cat C

Mental Health Medications

ANTI-ANXIETY AGENTS

DIAZEPAM

(dye-az-e-pam)

(Valium)

Side Effects

Dizziness
Drowsiness
Pain at IM site

Nursing Considerations

Management of anxiety and treatment of alcohol withdrawal
PO: onset 1–2 hours, peak 1/2–4 hours
IM: onset 15–30 minutes, slow, erratic absorption
IV: onset 1–5 minutes, duration 15–60 minutes
Use caution with activities requiring alertness until response to med is known
Abrupt stop may lead to withdrawal: insomnia, irritability, nervousness, tremors
Avoid alcohol, other CNS depressants
Tablets may be crushed and taken with food or fluids for ease of swallowing
Rx C = IV; Preg Cat D

ANTI-ANGINALS

ISOSORBIDE MONONITRATE

(eye-soe-sor-bide)

(Ismo)

Side Effects

Dizziness, postural hypotension
Vascular headache, flushing
Drowsiness
Nausea

Nursing Considerations

Treatment/prophylaxis of angina pectoris, CHF
PO: 1 hour before food or 2 hours after meals for maximum absorption, but taking with food may reduce or eliminate headache
Chewable tablet: chew well, hold in mouth for 2 minutes before swallowing
Sublingual: dissolve under tongue, do not eat, drink, talk, or smoke during use, go to ED if pain not relieved in 15 minutes
Avoid changing positions (lying/sitting/standing) rapidly
Use caution in potentially hazardous activities until stabilized
Avoid alcohol, smoking, strenuous exercise in hot environment
Wear medical identification tag
Rx; Preg Cat C

Mental Health Medications

ANTI-ANXIETY AGENTS

CHLORDIAZEPOXIDE

(klor-dye-az-e-pox-ide)

(Librium)

ANTI-ANGINALS

NITROGLYCERIN

(nye-troe-gli-ser-in)

(Nitro-dur, Transderm-Nitro, Nitrol/Nitrostat, Nitrotab)

Side Effects

Dizziness, headache,
Stimulation, insomnia, nervousness
Light-headedness, numbness
Nausea, diarrhea, constipation
Tachycardia, palpitations

Nursing Considerations

Management of anxiety disorders
Onset 7–10 days, optimum effect may take 3–4 weeks
Use caution with activities requiring alertness until response to med is known
Avoid alcohol, other CNS depressants
Caution when changing positions, because fainting may occur, esp. in elderly
Drowsiness may worsen at beginning of treatment
Rx; Preg Cat B

Side Effects

Transient headache

Nursing Considerations

Treatment/prophylaxis of angina pectoris; IV used for control of BP during surgery and CHF associated with acute MI

Sustained release: take every 6 to 12 hours on an empty stomach; onset 20–45 minutes, duration 3–8 hours

Sublingual: patient sitting/lying should let tablet dissolve under tongue and not swallow saliva; onset 1–3 minutes, duration 30 minutes

Spray: hold cannister vertically, spray on tongue, close mouth immediately, not inhale spray; onset 2 minutes, duration 30–60 minutes

IV: use infusion pump and special non-PVC tubing; onset 1–2 minutes, duration 3–5 minutes

Ointment: spread on skin in thin uniform layer; onset 30–60 minutes, duration 2–12 hours

Transdermal: apply to clean hairless area; rotate sites; onset 30–60 minutes, duration 12–24 hours

Go to ED if pain not relieved with 3 tablets in 15 minutes

Wear medical identification tag

Rx; Preg Cat C

Mental Health Medications

ANTI-ANXIETY AGENTS

BUSPIRONE

(byoo-spye-one)

(BuSpar)

ANTI-ARRHYTHMICS

AMIODARONE HCL

(am-ee-oh-da-rone)

(Cordarone, Pacerone)

KAPLAN

Side Effects

Dizziness, drowsiness

Orthostatic hypotension

Blurred vision

Nursing Considerations

Management of anxiety, panic disorders, premenstrual dysphoric disorders

Onset 30 minutes, peak 1–2 hours, duration 4–6 hours

Full therapeutic response takes 2 to 3 days

May be taken with food

May be habit forming; do not take for longer than 4 months unless directed

Memory impairment is a sign of long-term use

Do not stop drug abruptly

Drowsiness may worsen at beginning of treatment

Rx; Preg Cat D

Side Effects

- Dizziness, fatigue, malaise
- Corneal microdeposits
- Bradycardia, hypotension
- Nausea, vomiting
- Anorexia, constipation
- Photosensitivity
- Neurologic dysfunction

Nursing Considerations

- Management of ventricular arrhythmias unresponsive to less toxic agents
- IV: continuous cardiac monitoring
- Assess for signs of pulmonary toxicity: rales/crackles, decreased breath sounds, pleuritic friction rub, fatigue, dyspnea, cough, pleuritic pain, fever
- Neurotoxicity (ataxia, muscle weakness, tingling or numbness in fingers or toes, uncontrolled movements, tremors) common during initial therapy
- Side effects may not appear until several days, weeks or years and may persist for several months after stopping med
- Teach patient to check radial pulse
- Use sunscreen and protective clothing to prevent photosensitivity
- Rx; Preg Cat D

ANTI-ANXIETY AGENTS

ALPRAZOLAM

(al-pray-zoe-lam)

(Xanax)

LIDOCAINE HCL

(lye-doe-kane)

(Xylocaine)

Side Effects

Weight loss

Insomnia, irritability

Nervousness

Arrhythmias, tachycardia

Nursing Considerations

Management of hypothyroidism, myxedema coma, thyroid hormone replacement

PO: peak 1–3 weeks, duration 1–3 weeks

IV: onset 6–8 hours, peak 24 hours

PO: take at same time daily to maintain blood level; take on empty stomach

Do not switch brands unless directed

Avoid OTC meds with iodine and iodized salt, soybeans, tofu, turnips, some seafood, some bread

Drug is not a cure but controls symptoms and treatment is lifelong

Rx; Preg Cat A

Side Effects

- Hypotension, tremors
- Double vision
- Tinnitus
- Confusion, blurred vision
- Drowsiness, dizziness
- Twitching, convulsions
- Respiratory depression/arrest
- Bradycardia

Nursing Considerations

- Used for premature ventricular contractions
- Give oxygen; have resuscitation equipment available
- IV: use infusion pump; patient on cardiac monitor
- Check BUN, creatinine
- Rx; Preg Cat B

Hormones/Synthetic Substitutes/Modifiers

THYROID HORMONES

LEVOTHYROXINE (T4)

(lee-voe-thye-rox-een)

(Synthroid, Levothroid)

Cardiovascular Medications

ANTI-ARRHYTHMICS

PROCAINAMIDE

(proe-kane-a-mide)

(Procanbid, Pronestyl)

KAPLAN

Side Effects

Nausea, diarrhea
Bone pain and tenderness

Nursing Considerations

Treatment of Paget's disease, used with total hip replacement and spinal cord injury, hypercalemia of cancer
PO: onset 1 month, duration 1 year
IV: onset 24 hours, peak 3 days, duration 11 days
Take on empty stomach with calcium and Vitamin D but not within 2 hours of med
Contact clinician if sudden onset of unexpected pain, restricted mobility, heat over bone
Rx; Preg Cat B (oral) C (IV)

Side Effects

- Hypotension
- Bradycardia
- Fever, rash
- Nausea and vomiting
- Dizziness
- Neutropenia

Nursing Considerations

- Management of life-threatening ventricular dysrhythmias
- IV: use infusion pump; monitor BP q 5 to 15 minutes; on cardiac monitor; keep pt. recumbent
- IV: monitor CBC, blood levels, I&O, daily weight
- PO: best absorption on empty stomach, may take with food to decrease GI upset
- Take at equal intervals around the clock
- Teach patient to check radial pulse
- Avoid caffeine
- Rx; Preg Cat C

Hormones/Synthetic Substitutes/Modifiers

PARATHYROID AGENTS (CALCIUM REGULATORS)

ETIDRONATE

(eh-tih-droe-nate)

(Didronel)

ANTI-ARRHYTHMICS

QUINIDINE

(kwin-i-deen)

(Quinaglute)

Side Effects

Weakness
Diarrhea, abdominal pain
Bone pain

Nursing Considerations

Treatment of osteoporosis in postmenopausal women and for Paget's disease
Onset: within days, peak 30 days, duration up to 16 months
Take in AM before food or other meds with full glass of water; remain upright for 30 minutes
Take with calcium and Vitamin D if instructed by clinician
Rx; Preg Cat C

Side Effects

Anemia
Hypotension
Headache
Heart block
Tinnitus, fever
Nausea, vomiting, diarrhea

Nursing Considerations

Used for atrial or ventricular arrhythmias
May increase toxicity for digitalis
Monitor liver function tests and I and 0
Check apical pulse and BP
Monitor EKG and BP
Avoid changing positions (lying/sitting/standing) rapidly
Avoid use with alcohol, caffeine
Patient should wear medical information tag
Rx; Preg Cat C

Hormones/Synthetic Substitutes/Modifiers

BONE RESORPTION INHIBITORS

RISEDRONATE

(riss-ed-roe-nate)

(Actonel)

ANTI-ARRHYTHMICS

SOTATOL

(soe-ta-lole)

(Betapace)

Side Effects

Esophageal ulceration

Nursing Considerations

Treatment of osteoporosis in postmenopausal women and in men, Paget's disease

Onset: 1 month, peak 3–6 months, duration 3 weeks to 7 months

Take in AM before food or other meds with full glass of water; remain upright for 30 minutes

If dose missed, skip dose, do not double doses or take later in the day

Take with calcium and Vitamin D if instructed by clinician

Rx; Preg Cat C

Side Effects

Fatigue
Weakness
Impotence

Nursing Considerations

Management of life-threatening ventricular arrhythmias
Teach patient to check radial pulse, if less than 50, hold med and contact clinician
Change positions (sitting/standing/lying) slowly
Avoid activities that require alertness until drug response known
Contact clinician if slow pulse, difficulty breathing, wheezing, cold hands and feet, dizziness, confusion, depression, rash, fever, sore throat, unusual bleeding or bruising
Rx; Preg Cat B

Hormones/Synthetic Substitutes/Modifiers

BONE RESORPTION INHIBITORS

ALENDRONATE

(al-en-drone-ate)

(Fosamax)

ANTI-HYPERTENSIVES

BISOPROLOL

(bis-<u>oh</u>-pro-lole)

(Zebeta)

Side Effects

Dizziness
Nausea, vomiting, diarrhea
Abdominal pain
Tooth staining

Nursing Considerations

Treatment of urinary tract infections
Take with food or milk
Avoid alcohol
Two daily doses if urine output is high or patient has diabetes
Drug may turn urine rust-yellow to brown
Rx; Preg Cat B

Side Effects

GI upset
Fatigue
Weakness

Nursing Considerations

Treatment of mild to moderate hypertension
Peak: 2–4 hours
Therapeutic response in 1 to 2 weeks
Do not stop med abruptly, may precipitate angina
Do not use OTC meds with stimulants, such as nasal decongestants, OTC cold meds, unless directed
Avoid alcohol, smoking, sodium intake
Contact clinician if signs of CHF: difficulty breathing, night cough, swelling of extremities
Rx, Preg Cat C

Genitourinary Medications

URINARY ANTI-INFECTIVES

NITROFURANTOIN

(nye-troe-fyoor-an-toyn)

(Furadantin, Macrobid, Macrodantin)

Cardiovascular Medications

ANTI-HYPERTENSIVES

CLONIDINE PATCH

(kloe-ni-deen)

(Catapres)

Side Effects

GI upset

Kidney and liver toxicity

Nursing Considerations

Treatment of urinary tract irritation, often paired with urinary anti-infective

Can crush tablets for ease of swallowing; can take with food or milk to decrease GI upset

Inform patient that urine will be bright orange/red; may stain clothes or contact lens

Monitor for signs of hepatoxicity: dark urine, clay-colored stools, jaundice, itching, abdominal pain, fever, diarrhea

Rx/OTC; Preg Cat B

Side Effects

Drowsiness, sedation
Dry mouth
Dizziness
Headache
Severe rebound hypertension

Nursing Considerations

Treatment of hypertension, severe cancer pain (in combination with opiates)
Avoid changing positions (lying/sitting/standing) rapidly
Avoid use with alcohol, CNS depressants
Avoid high sodium foods (canned soups, lunch meats, cheese)
Use caution in potentially hazardous activities
Avoid alcohol, smoking, strenuous exercise in hot environment
Apply patch to non-hairy area (upper outer arm, anterior chest), rotate sites, do not apply to scarred or irritated area
Wear medical identification tag
Rx; Preg Cat C

URINARY ANALGESICS

PHENAZOPYRIDINE HCL

(fen-az-oh-peer-i-deen)

(Azo, Pyridium)

Side Effects

Decreased libido
Impotence
Breast tenderness
Decreased volume of ejaculate

Nursing Considerations

Treatment of benign prostatic hyperplasia (BPH) by Proscar, male hair loss by Propecia
May be taken without regard for food
Pregnant women should avoid contact with crushed drug or patient's semen; may adversely affect developing male fetus
Full therapeutic effect: Propecia may require 3 months, Proscar may require 6–12 months
Rx; Preg Cat X

(Apresoline)

(hye-dral-a-zeen)

HYDRALAZINE HCL

ANTI-HYPERTENSIVES

Side Effects

Headache
Palpitations, tachycardia, angina
Edema
Lupus erythematosus-like syndrome
Nausea, vomiting, diarrhea
Anorexia
Tremors
Dizziness
Anxiety

Nursing Considerations

Used to treat essential hypertension
PO: give with meals to enhance absorption
Observe mental status
Check for weight gain, edema
Avoid changing positions (lying/sitting/standing) rapidly
Contact clinician if chest pain, severe fatigue, fever, muscle or joint pain

TESTOSTERONE INHIBITORS

FINASTERIDE

(fin-as-the-ride)

(Proscar, Propecia)

HYDROCHLOROTHIAZIDE/LISINOPRIL

(hye-droe-klor-oh-thye-a-zide)

(Prinizide, Zestoretic)

Side Effects

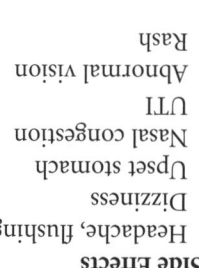

Headache, flushing
Dizziness
Upset stomach
Nasal congestion
UTI
Abnormal vision
Rash

Nursing Considerations

Treatment of erectile dysfunction
Take approximately 1 hour before sexual activity
Do not use more than once a day
Tablets may be split
High-fat meal will reduce absorption; better absorption on empty stomach
Never use with nitrates; could have fatal fall in blood pressure
Notify clinician if erection lasts longer than 4 hours
Rx; Preg Cat B

Side Effects

- Headache
- Dizziness
- Hypotension
- Tachycardia
- Nausea, vomiting, diarrhea
- Fatigue

Nursing Considerations

- Used to treat essential hypertension
- Avoid changing positions (lying/sitting/standing) rapidly
- May take without regard to food
- Avoid high Na^+ foods (canned soups, lunch meats, cheese)
- Avoid high K^+ foods (bananas, citrus fruits, raisins)

Genitourinary Medications

ANTI-IMPOTENCE

SILDANAFIL CITRATE

(sil-den-a-fill)

(Viagra)

MINOXIDIL

(mi-nox-i-dill)

(Loniten)

Side Effects

Anxiety, restlessness
Dizziness
Convulsions
Palpitations, tachycardia
Nausea, vomiting
Anorexia
Drowsiness, blurred vision
Dry mouth
Mydriasis

Nursing Considerations

Antispasmodic treatment of neurogenic bladder
Take on an empty stomach
Avoid alcohol, other CNS depressants
Avoid activities requiring alertness until med response is known
Decreased ability to perspire means avoid strenuous activity in warm weather
Wear sunglasses in bright sunlight to prevent photophobia
Rx; Preg Cat B

Side Effects

Edema
Increase in body hair

Nursing Considerations

Limited to treat severe symptomatic hypertension or uncontrolled by other means
Teach patient to take radial pulse
Check for weight gain, edema
Rx; Preg Cat C

ANTICHOLINERGICS

OXYBUTYNIN CHLORIDE

(ox-i-byoo-ti-nin)

(Ditropan)

ANTI-HYPERTENSIVES

RESERPINE

(re-ser-peen)

(Serpasil)

Side Effects

Abdominal pain (high doses only)
Nausea, diarrhea
Stomach cramps

Nursing Considerations

Used to replace or supplement naturally occurring enzymes, contains lipase, amylase, and protease
Take with 8 ounces of water and food, swallow right away, sit up when taking
Do not crush or break enteric-coated capsules
Do not use if sensitivity or allergy to pork
Stools will be foul-smelling and frothy
Rx; Preg Cat C

Side Effects

Depression
Orthostatic hypotension
Nasal stuffiness
Bradycardia

Nursing Considerations

Treatment of hypertension
Seriousness of side effects and availability of newer, less risky medications have led to less use of this medication
Caution needed to assess despondency; otherwise continued therapy could lead to suicide
Caution needed with a history of gallstones, to prevent biliary colic
Caution needed with a history of renal insufficiency, to avoid decreased renal tissue perfusion
Caution needed with ulcerative colitis or acute peptic ulcer disease, to avoid increased GI motility
Rx; Preg Cat NA

Gastrointestinal Medications

PANCREATIC ENZYMES

PANCRELIPASE

(pan-kree-ly-payz)

(Pancrease, Viokase)

Cardiovascular Medications

ANTILIPEMIC AGENTS

COLESTIPOL

(koe-les-ti-pole)

(Colestid)

Side Effects

Anorexia

Nausea, vomiting, diarrhea

Nursing Considerations

Do not crush or break enteric-coated capsules

Do not use if sensitivity or allergy to pork

Rx; Preg Cat C

Side Effects

- Constipation
- Abdominal pain
- Nausea
- Decreased vitamin A, D, K

Nursing Considerations

- Used to lower cholesterol levels, digitalis toxicity, biliary obstruction pruritus, and diarrhea
- Take other meds 1 hour before or 4 hours after this med to avoid poor absorption
- Mix granules in applesauce or liquid, do not take dry, let stand for 2 minutes
- Monitor for hypoprothrombinemia: bleeding gums, tarry stools, hematuria, bruising
- Rx; Preg Cat B

Gastrointestinal Medications

PANCREATIC ENZYMES

PANCREATIN

(pān-kree-a-tin)

ANTILIPEMIC AGENTS

GEMFIBROZIL

(jem-fi-broe-zil)

Side Effects

Nausea, vomiting
Abdominal cramps

Nursing Considerations

Used for chronic constipation
PO: Take with water or fruit juice to counteract sweet taste
Rx

Side Effects

Abdominal pain, diarrhea
GI upset

Nursing Considerations

Used to lower cholesterol levels
Take one-half hour before meals
Check CBC and liver function tests
PO: take 30 minutes before morning and evening meals
May stop if no improvement in 3 months
Rx; Preg Cat C

Gastrointestinal Medications

LAXATIVES

LACTULOSE SYRUP

(lak-tyoo-lose)

(Cephulac, Duphalac, Enulose)

ANTILIPEMIC AGENTS

LOVASTATIN

(loh-vah-stat-in)

(Mevacor)

Side Effects

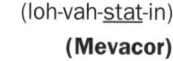

CNS stimulation
Hypertension
Palpitations
Drowsiness

Nursing Considerations

Short-term treatment of obesity
PO: hydrochloride form duration is 4 hours
PO: resin complex form duration is 12–14 hours
Take 30 minutes before meals or as a single dose before breakfast or 10–14 hours before bedtime
Avoid activities requiring alertness until response is known
Avoid alcohol, other CNS depressants
Contact clinician if chest pain, decreased exercise tolerance, fainting or lower extremity swelling
Controlled Substance Schedule IV; Preg Cat NA

Side Effects

Flatus, constipation
Abdominal pain, nausea, diarrhea, GI upset
Heart burn
Muscle cramps
Dizziness
Headache
Tremor
Blurred vision
Rash, pruritus

Nursing Considerations

Used to lower cholesterol levels, primary and secondary prevention of coronary events
Use sunscreen to prevent photosensitivity reactions
Schedule liver function tests every 1 to 2 months during the first 1 1/2 years
Onset 2 weeks, peak 4–6 weeks, duration 6 weeks
Take with food, absorption is reduced by 30 percent on an empty stomach
Contact clinician if unexplained muscle pain, tenderness or weakness, esp. if with fever or malaise
Rx; Preg Cat X

APPETITE SUPPRESSANTS

PHENTERMINE

(fēn-ter-meen)

NIACIN

(nye-a-sin)

(Niacor for immediate release; Niaspan for sustained release)

Side Effects

Headache
Anorexia
Nausea, vomiting, diarrhea
Rashes
Fever

Nursing Considerations

Used for treatment of inflammatory bowel diseases and arthritis
PO: Take with food to decrease GI upset
Encourage fluids to decrease crystalization in kidneys
May permanently stain contact lens yellow
May cause orange-yellow urine and skin, which is not significant
Wear sunscreen and protective clothing to prevent photosensitivity reactions
Rx; Preg Cat B

Side Effects

Headache
Nausea
Postural hypotension

Nursing Considerations

Treatment of pellagra, hyperlipidemias, peripheral vascular disease
Take with meals to reduce GI upset, can add 325 mg ASA 1/2 hour before dose to reduce flushing
Flushing will occur several hours after med taken, will decrease over 2 weeks
Avoid changing positions (sitting/standing/lying) rapidly
Rx/OTC; Preg Cat C

Gastrointestinal Medications

ANTI-ULCER MEDICATIONS

SULFASALAZINE

(sul-fah-sal-ah-zeen)

(Azulfidine)

NICOTINIC ACID

(nih-koh-tin-ick)

(Slo-Niacin, Vitamin B)

Side Effects

Constipation

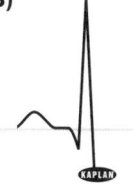

Nursing Considerations

Short-term treatment (less than 8 weeks) of duodenal ulcers

PO: 1 hour before meals or 2 hours after meals and at hs with full glass of water

Do not chew tablets

Do not use antacids within half an hour of med

Encourage 8 to 10 glasses of fluid per day

Avoid use with smoking

Rx; Preg Cat B

Side Effects

Headache
Nausea
Postural hypotension

Nursing Considerations

Treatment of pellagra, hyperlipidemias, peripheral vascular disease
Take with meals to reduce GI upset, can add 325 mg ASA 1/2 hour before dose to reduce flushing
Flushing will occur several hours after med taken, will decrease over 2 weeks
Avoid changing positions (sitting/standing/lying) rapidly
Rx/OTC; Preg Cat C

Gastrointestinal Medications

ANTI-ULCER MEDICATIONS

SUCRALFATE

(soo-kral-fate)

(Carafate)

ANTILIPEMIC AGENTS

PRAVASTATIN

(pra-va-sta-tin)

(Pravachol)

Side Effects

Dizziness (esp. in elderly)
Drowsiness
Headache

Nursing Considerations

Used to inhibit gastric acid secretion
Take with or immediately following meals
Do not take antacids within 1 hour before or after
Do not smoke; it interferes with healing and drug's effectiveness
Avoid alcohol, ASA, and caffeine which increase stomach acid
Rx/OTC; Preg Cat B

Side Effects

Abdominal cramps, flatus
Constipation, diarrhea
Heartburn

Nursing Considerations

Treatment of hypercholesterolemia, apolipoprotein B (apo B), risk reduction of recurrent MI, atherosclerosis
Schedule liver function tests semiannually
Take without regard to food
Contact clinician if unexplained muscle pain, tenderness or weakness, esp. if with fever or malaise
Rx; Preg Cat X

Gastrointestinal Medications

ANTI-ULCER MEDICATIONS

RANITIDINE

(ra-nit-i-deen)

(Zantac)

Cardiovascular Medications

ANTILIPEMIC AGENTS

SIMVASTATIN

(sim-va-sta-tin)

(Zocor)

Side Effects

Headache
Dizziness
Nausea, vomiting, diarrhea
Constipation, flatulence
Rash
Back pain

Nursing Considerations

Used for treatment of GERD and duodenal ulcers
Take on an empty stomach before eating
Swallow tablets whole; do not crush, chew or split tablets
Avoid alcohol, NSAIDs and ASA; may increase gastric upset
Rx; Preg Cat B

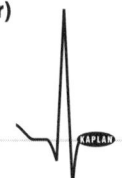

Side Effects

Eye lens opacities
Liver dysfunction

Nursing Considerations

Treatment of hypercholesterolemia, hypertriglyceridemia, hyperlipoproteinemias, coronary artery disease
Have eye exam before, 1 month after, and then annually after starting med, lens opacities may occur
Schedule liver function tests semiannually
Take without regard to food
Contact clinician if unexplained muscle pain, tenderness or weakness, esp. if with fever or malaise
Rx; Preg Cat X

ANTI-ULCER MEDICATIONS

RABEPRAZOLE

(rah-bep-rah-zole)

(Aciphex)

BETA BLOCKERS

ATENOLOL

(a-<u>ten</u>-oh-lole)

(Tenormin, Tenoretic is combination with Chlorthalidone)

Side Effects

Abdominal pain
Diarrhea (13 percent)
Miscarriage

Nursing Considerations

Prevention of gastric ulcers during NSAIA therapy
Take with meals and at bedtime
Avoid taking magnesium antacids within 2 hours
Notify clinician if diarrhea lasts more than 1 week
Notify clinician if black, tarry stools or severe abdominal pain
Rx; Preg Cat X

Side Effects

- Bradycardia, cold extremities
- Postural hypotension
- Bronchospasm in overdose
- 2nd or 3rd degree heart block
- Cold extremities
- Insomnia, fatigue
- Dizziness
- Mental changes
- Nausea, diarrhea

Nursing Considerations

- Used in treatment of hypertension, MI (IV use), prophylaxis of angina
- Masks signs of hypoglycemia in diabetics
- Teach patient how to take radial pulse
- Check pulse, if less than 50 beats per minute, hold the med and contact clinician
- PO: Take before meals, at bedtime
- Tablet may be crushed or swallowed whole
- Do not stop abruptly; taper over 2 weeks
- Rx; Preg Cat D

Gastrointestinal Medications

ANTI-ULCER MEDICATIONS

MISOPROSTOL

(mis-oh-prost-ole)

(Cytotec)

CARVEDILOL

(kar-ved-i-lole)

(Coreg)

Side Effects

Dizziness
Diarrhea

Nursing Considerations

Used for treatment of GERD and ulcers
PO: Take no more than 30 minutes before meals. Capsules may be opened and sprinkled on food (applesauce, pudding, cottage cheese, yogurt) and swallowed immediately.
Can use with antacids
Do not crush or chew capsule contents.
To give with NG tube in place, open the capsule and mix with orange, apple or tomato juice, instill through NG tube and flush with additional juice to clear tube
Report severe diarrhea
Rx: Preg Cat B

Side Effects

Dizziness
Diarrhea
Postural hypotension
Impotence
Hyperglycemia

Nursing Considerations

Used in treatment of hypertension, CHF
PO: Take with food
Tablet may be crushed or swallowed whole
Do not stop abruptly; taper over 1 to 2 weeks
Rx; Preg Cat C

ANTI-ULCER MEDICATIONS

LANSOPRAZOLE

(lan-sō-prey-zohl)

(Prevacid)

METOPROLOL SUCCINATE

(meh-toe-proe-lole)

(ToprolXL, the sustained release form)

Side Effects

Headache
Dizziness
Constipation
Blood dyscrasias

Nursing Considerations

Treatment of duodenal and gastric ulcers, gastroesophageal reflux disease, heartburn
PO: onset 30–60 minutes, peak 1–3 hours, duration 6–12 hours
IV: onset immediate, peak 30–60 minutes, duration 8–15 hours
Signs of blood dyscrasia: bleeding, bruising, fatigue, malaise, poor healing
OTC, Rx; Preg Cat B

Side Effects

Bradycardia, palpitations
Hypotension
Congestive heart failure
Depression
Insomnia
Dizziness
Nausea, vomiting, diarrhea

Nursing Considerations

Used in treatment of hypertension, MI (IV use), prophylaxis of angina
Teach patient how to take radial pulse
Check pulse, if less than 50 beats per minute, hold the med and contact clinician
PO: May be taken with food
Tablet must be swallowed whole
Do not stop abruptly; taper over 2 weeks; may precipitate angina
Do not use OTC products (nasal decongestants, cold preparations) unless directed by prescriber
Rx; Preg Cat C

Gastrointestinal Medications

ANTI-ULCER MEDICATIONS

FAMOTIDINE

(fa-moe-ti-deen)

(Pepcid)

METOPROLOL TARTRATE

(meh-toe-proe-lole)

(Lopressor, the immediate release form)

Side Effects

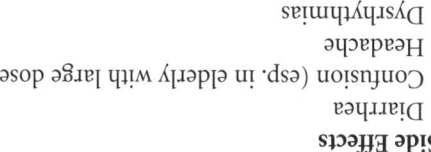

- Diarrhea
- Confusion (esp. in elderly with large doses)
- Headache
- Dysrhythmias

Nursing Considerations

- Reduces gastric acid secretions by 50–80%
- May be taken without regard to meals
- Avoid antacids 1 hour before or after dose
- Do not use OTC for more than 2 weeks unless medically supervised
- Monitor liver enzymes and blood counts
- OTC/Rx; Preg Cat B

Side Effects

Bradycardia, palpitations
Hypotension
Congestive heart failure
Depression
Insomnia
Dizziness
Nausea, vomiting, diarrhea
Constipation

Nursing Considerations

Used in treatment of hypertension, MI (IV use), prophylaxis of angina
Teach patient how to take radial pulse
Check pulse, if less than 50 beats per minute, hold the med and contact clinician
PO: Take on an empty stomach, before meals, at bedtime
Tablet may be crushed or swallowed whole
Do not stop abruptly; taper over 2 weeks; may precipitate angina
Do not use OTC products (nasal decongestants, cold preparations) unless directed by prescriber
Rx; Preg Cat C

Gastrointestinal Medications

ANTI-ULCER MEDICATIONS

CIMETIDINE

(sye-met-ih-deen)

(Tagamet)

Side Effects

Belching

Rectal flatus

Nursing Considerations

Helps disperse gas pockets in GI system, does not decrease gas production

Take after meals, at bedtime

Shake suspension well before pouring

Tablets must be chewed

Rx/OTC; Preg Cat C

BETA BLOCKERS

PROPRANOLOL HCL

(proe-pran-oh-lole)

(Inderal)

Side Effects

- Weakness
- Hypotension
- Bronchospasm
- Bradycardia
- Depression

Nursing Considerations

Used in treatment of stable angina, hypertension, dysrhythmias, migraine, prophylaxis MI, essential tremor, alcohol withdrawal

Teach patient how to take radial pulse

Check pulse, if less than 50 beats per minute, hold the med and contact clinician

PO: Take with full glass of water at the same time each day

Do not open, chew, crush extended release capsule

Do not stop abruptly; taper over 2 weeks; may precipitate life-threatening dysrhythmias

Do not use aluminum-containing antacid; may decrease absorption

Rx; Preg Cat C

Gastrointestinal Medications

ANTIFLATULENTS

SIMETHICONE

(si-meth-i-kone)

Cardiovascular Medications

BETA BLOCKERS

SOTATOL

(soe-ta-lole)

(Betapace)

Side Effects

Drowsiness
Dizziness
Constipation
Urinary retention
Dry mouth

Nursing Considerations

Management of motion sickness, rhinitis, allergy symptoms, sedation, nausea, pre and post-operative sedation
PO: onset 20 minutes, duration 4–6 hours
Take 1/2–1 hour before traveling
Avoid activities requiring alertness
Avoid alcohol, other CNS depressants
Rx; Preg Cat C

Side Effects

Fatigue
Weakness
Impotence

Nursing Considerations

Management of life-threatening ventricular arrhythmias
Teach patient to check radial pulse, if less than 50, hold med and contact clinician
Change positions (sitting/standing/lying) slowly
Avoid activities that require alertness until drug response known
Contact clinician if slow pulse, difficulty breathing, wheezing, cold hands and feet, dizziness, confusion, depression, rash, fever, sore throat, unusual bleeding or bruising
Rx; Preg Cat B

Gastrointestinal Medications

ANTIEMETICS

PROMETHAZINE

(Phenergan)

DILTIAZEM HCL

(dil-tye-a-zem)

(Cardizem, Dilacor, Tiamate, Tiazac)

Side Effects

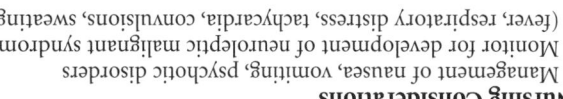

Orthostatic hypotension
Blurred vision
Dry eyes, dry mouth
Constipation
Drowsiness
Photosensitivity

Nursing Considerations

Management of nausea, vomiting, psychotic disorders
Monitor for development of neuroleptic malignant syndrome (fever, respiratory distress, tachycardia, convulsions, sweating, hypertension or hypotension, pallor, tiredness, severe muscle stiffness, loss of bladder control). Notify clinician immediately
PO: Take with food
Do not crush or break sustained release capsules
IM: inject slowly, deeply into gluteal UOQ; keep patient lying down for 30 minutes
Use caution with potentially hazardous activities
Avoid changing positions (lying/sitting/standing) rapidly
Wear sunscreen and protective clothing to prevent photosensitivity reactions
Check CBC and liver functions with prolonged use
Rx; Preg Cat C

Side Effects

Hypotension, dizziness
Edema
Nausea, constipation
Rash
Headache
Fatigue, drowsiness

Nursing Considerations

Management of angina, hypertension, vasospasm, atrial fibrillation, flutter, paroxysmal supraventricular tachycardia
Reduces workload of left ventricle, coronary vasodilator
Monitor blood pressure during dosage adjustments
PO: Take on an empty stomach, with a full glass of water
Teach patient how to take radial pulse and keep records of pulse rate
Avoid hazardous activities until stabilized on drug
Rx; Preg Cat C

Gastrointestinal Medications

ANTIEMETICS

PROCHLORPERAZINE

(proe-klor-pair-a-zeen)

(Compazine)

FELODIPINE

(fe-loe-di-peen)

(Plendil)

Side Effects

Drowsiness
Restlessness
Lassitude
Headache
Sleeplessness
Dry mouth
Anxiety

Nursing Considerations

Prevention of nausea, vomiting induced by chemotherapy, radiation, delayed gastric emptying, GERD
Used with tube feeding to decrease residual and risk of aspiration
PO: Take half an hour to an hour before meals or procedures
IV: Inject slowly over 1 to 2 minutes; infuse over 15 minutes
Use caution with potentially hazardous activities
Avoid alcohol and other CNS depressants
Rx; Preg Cat B

Side Effects

Dysrhythmia
Headache
Fatigue

Nursing Considerations

Used in treatment of essential hypertension, angina
Do not adjust dosage at intervals of less than 2 weeks
PO: Take without regard to meals
Do not open, chew, or crush extended release capsule
Do not use OTC products or alcohol unless directed by prescriber; limit caffeine
Rx; Preg Cat C

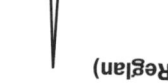

Gastrointestinal Medications

ANTIEMETICS

METOCLOPRAMIDE HCL

(met-oh-kloe-pra-mide)

(Reglan)

CALCIUM CHANNEL BLOCKERS

NIFEDIPINE

(nye-fed-i-peen)

(Adalat CC, Procardia XL)

Side Effects

Drowsiness
Dizziness

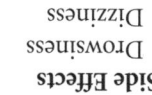

Nursing Considerations

Management of vertigo, motion sickness
Duration 8–14 hours
Take 1 hour before traveling
Avoid activities requiring alertness
Avoid alcohol, other CNS depressants
OTC, Rx;

Side Effects

Orthostatic hypotension

Nursing Considerations

Used in treatment of hypertension, angina

Avoid changing positions (sitting/standing/lying) rapidly

PO: Take on an empty stomach; onset 20 minutes, peak 1/2 hour–6 hours, duration 6–8 hours

PO of extended release capsule: do not open, chew, crush; can take without regard to meals; duration of 24 hours, shell may appear in stools, but is insignificant

Do not use OTC products or alcohol unless directed by prescriber; limit caffeine

Rx; Preg Cat C

ANTIEMETICS

MECLIZINE

(mek-li-zeen)

(Antivert, Bonine)

CALCIUM CHANNEL BLOCKERS

VERAPAMIL HCL

(ver-ap-a-mill)

(Calan, Isoptin, Covera)

Side Effects

Nausea, vomiting
Abdominal pain/distention
Dizziness
Drowsiness
Dry mouth

Nursing Considerations

Used for control of diarrhea, including diarrhea in travelers
Take with a full glass of H_2O
Encourage 6 to 8 glasses of fluid per day
Use caution with potentially hazardous activities
If abdominal distention in acute ulcerative colitis, stop med
Avoid use with alcohol, CNS depressants
Follow clear liquid or bland diet until diarrhea subsides
Do not use OTC if fever over 101° F (38° C) or if bloody diarrhea
Rx/OTC; Preg Cat B

Side Effects

- Edema
- Nausea, constipation
- Headache
- Drowsiness

Nursing Considerations

- Management of chronic stable angina, sysrhythmias, hypertension, supraventricular tachycardia, atrial flutter or fibrillation
- PO: Take before meals, except sustained release to be taken with food
- Do not open, chew, crush sustained or extended release capsule
- Increased hypotensive effects with grapefruit juice
- Teach patient how to take radial pulse and keep records of pulse rate
- Avoid hazardous activities until stabilized on drug
- Do not use OTC products or alcohol unless directed by prescriber; limit caffeine
- Rx; Preg Cat C

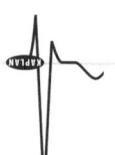

Gastrointestinal Medications

ANTIDIARRHEALS

LOPERAMIDE HCL

(loe-per-a-mide)

(Imodium)

DIGITALIS GLYCOSIDES

DIGOXIN

(di-jox-in)

(Lanoxin)

Side Effects

Confusion, stimulation in elderly
Dry mouth, constipation
Urinary retention, hesitancy
Palpitations
Blurred vision

Nursing Considerations

Treatment of peptic ulcer, other GI disorders, other spastic disorders, urinary incontinence
PO: onset 20–30 minutes, duration 4–6 hours
IM, IV, subQ: onset 2–3 minutes, duration 4–6 hours
Avoid activities requiring alertness until stabilized on med
Avoid alcohol, other CNS depressants
Use sunglasses to prevent photophobia
Rx; Preg Cat C

Side Effects

Headache
Hypotension

Nursing Considerations

Used in treatment of CHF, atrial fibrillation, flutter or tachycardia, cardiogenic shock
Check pulse, if less than 60 beats per minute (adult) or 90 beats per minute (infant), hold the med and contact clinician
PO: with or without food; may crush tablets and mix with food/fluids
Do not open, chew, crush capsule
Contact clinician if loss of appetite, lower stomach pain, diarrhea, weakness, drowsiness, headache, blurred or yellow vision, rash, depression
Eat a sodium-restricted and potassium-rich (bananas, orange juice) diet to keep potassium level normal
Avoid OTC meds and herbals, many adverse interactions may occur
Rx; Preg Cat C

Gastrointestinal Medications

ANTICHOLINERGICS

HYOSCYAMINE

(hye-oh-sye-a-meen)

(Anaspaz, Gastrosed)

LOOP DIURETICS

BUMETANIDE

(byoo-met-a-nide)

(Bumex)

Side Effects

Drowsiness
Blurred vision

Nursing Considerations

Used for treatment of irritable bowel syndrome
Take 30 minutes before meals and at bedtime
Use caution with potentially hazardous activities
Rx; Preg Cat C

Side Effects

- Potassium depletion
- Electrolyte imbalance
- Hypovolemia
- Ototoxicity
- Hyperglycemia

Nursing Considerations

- Used in treatment of hypertension
- PO: diuresis onset 30-60 minutes, peak 1–2 hours, duration 3–6 hours
- IM: diuresis onset 40 minutes, peak 1–2 hours, duration 4–6 hours
- IV: diuresis onset 5 minutes, peak 15–30 minutes, duration 3–6 hours
- Weigh daily
- Do not take at bedtime to prevent nocturia
- Encourage potassium-containing foods
- Rx; Preg Cat C

Gastrointestinal Medications

ANTICHOLINERGICS

DICYCLOMINE HCL

(dye-sye-kloh-meen)

(Bentyl)

LOOP DIURETICS

FUROSEMIDE

(fur-oh-se-mide)

(Lasix)

Side Effects

Nausea

Nursing Considerations

Used as antacid and calcium supplement

May decrease effect of some antibiotics and other drugs due to impaired absorption, so separate administration times by 2 hours

Do not use if ventricular fibrillation or hypercalcemia

Use caution if taking cardiac glycoside or has sarcoidosis or renal or cardiac disease

Signs of hypercalcemia: nausea, vomiting, headache, confusion, anorexia

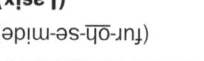

Side Effects

Hypotension
Hypokalemia
Hyperglycemia
Nausea
Polyuria
Rash, pruritus

Nursing Considerations

Used in treatment of pulmonary edema, and edema in other conditions
PO: diuresis onset 60 minutes, peak 1–2 hours, duration 6–8 hours
IV: diuresis onset 5 minutes, peak 1/2 hour, duration 2 hours
PO: take with food or milk to prevent GI upset, slightly lessened absorption, tablets may be crushed
Take early in the day to prevent nocturia and sleeplessness
Avoid changing positions (sitting/standing/lying) rapidly
Use sunscreen or protective clothing to prevent photosensitivity
Rx; Preg Cat C

Gastrointestinal Medications

ANTACIDS

CALCIUM CARBONATE

(Tums)

CLOPIDOGREL BISULFATE

(klo-pid-oh-grel)

(Plavix)

Side Effects

Mild constipation

Diarrhea

Increased urine pH levels

Hypophosphotemia

Nursing Considerations

Antacid with onset in 20 minutes and duration of 20 to 180 minutes

May decrease effect of antibiotics and other drugs, such as digoxin, phenothiazines, quinidine, salicylates due to impaired absorption, so separate administration times by 1 to 2 hours

Since low sodium content, used in patients on sodium restriction

If given with enteric-coated drugs, might have premature release in stomach; separate administration times by at least 1 hour

Shake suspension well and follow with small amount of water to facilitate passage

Contact clinician if signs of GI bleeding: tarry stools or coffee-grounds vomitus

Side Effects

GI bleeding
Nausea, vomiting, diarrhea, GI discomfort
Depression

Nursing Considerations

Used to reduce risk of stroke, MI, peripheral artery disease in high risk patients
Monitor blood studies in long-term therapy
Take with meals or just after to decrease gastric symptoms
Report signs of unusual bruising, bleeding; it may take longer to stop bleeding
Rx, Preg Cat B

Gastrointestinal Medications

ANTACIDS

ALUMINUM HYDROXIDE AND MAGNESIUM TRISILICATE

(Riopan)

PLATELET AGGREGATION INHIBITORS

DIPYRIDAMOLE

(dye-peer-id-a-mole)

(Persantine)

Side Effects

Constipation that may lead to impaction
Phosphate depletion

Nursing Considerations

Antacid with duration of effect of 20 to 180 minutes
Aluminum antacid compounds interfere with tetracycline absorption
Contact clinician if signs of GI bleeding: tarry stools or coffee-grounds vomitus
Shake suspension well and follow with small amount of milk or water to facilitate passage
Monitor long-term, high-dose use if on restricted sodium intake, due to high sodium content
If prolonged use, monitor for phosphate depletion: anorexia, malaise, and muscle weakness; can also lead to resorption of calcium and bone demineralization in uremia patients
Use may interfere with some imaging techniques
Because drug contains aluminum, used in renal failure to control hyperphosphatemia by binding with phosphate in the GI tract

Side Effects

- Headache
- Dizziness
- Nausea, vomiting
- Postural hypotension
- Weakness, fainting, syncope
- Rash

Nursing Considerations

Prevention of transient ischemic attacks, MIs, with warfarin in heart valves, with ASA in bypass grafts

PO: peak in 2 to 2 1/2 hours; duration 6 hours

PO: on an empty stomach, 1 hour before or 2 hours after meals with full glass of water

Full therapeutic response may take several months

IV: do not give undiluted, give over 4 minutes

Use caution with hazardous activities until stabilized on med

Avoid changing positions (sitting/standing/lying) rapidly

Rx; Preg Cat B

Gastrointestinal Medications

ANTACIDS

ALUMINUM HYDROXIDE GEL

(Amphojel)

PLATELET AGGREGATION INHIBITORS

TICLOPIDINE HCL

(ty-<u>cloe</u>-pi-deen)

(Ticlid)

Side Effects

Nausea, vomiting

Nursing Considerations

Acute management of severe hypoglycemia; facilitation of GI x-rays

IM for hypoglycemia: onset within 10 minutes, peak 30 minutes, duration 60-90 minutes

IV for hypoglycemia: onset within 10 minutes, peak 5 minutes, duration 60-90 minutes

SubQ for hypoglycemia: onset within 10 minutes, peak 30–45 minutes, duration 60–90 minutes

IV for GI x-rays: onset within 45 seconds, duration dose dependent of 9–25 minutes

IM for GI x-rays: onset within 8–10 minutes, duration dose dependent of 9–32 minutes

Rx, OTC; Preg Cat B

Side Effects

- Rash
- Diarrhea
- Bleeding

Nursing Considerations

- Prevention of stroke in high risk patients
- Monitor blood studies in long-term therapy
- Take with meals or just after to decrease gastric symptoms
- Monitor for signs of cholestasis (jaundice, dark urine, light-colored stools)
- Rx; Preg Cat B

Diabetic Medications

REVERSAL OF HYPOGLYCEMIA

GLUCAGON

(gloo-ka-gon)

(GlucaGen)

POTASSIUM-SPARING/COMBINATION DIURETICS

HYDROCHLOROTHIAZIDE/TRIAMTERENE

(hye-droe-klor-oh-thye-a-zide/trye-am-ter-een)

(Dyazide, Maxzide)

Side Effects

Hypoglycemia
Lipodystrophy

Nursing Considerations

Management of mild to moderate hyperglycemia in stabilized diabetics
Comes in 100 units per milliliter vial
Large crystals of insulin and a high content of size are responsible for the slow-acting properties
subQ: onset 4–8 hours, peak 10–30 hours, duration 36 hours or longer

Side Effects

Nausea, vomiting, diarrhea
Anemia

Nursing Considerations

Used in treatment of edema and hypertension
Diuresis onset 2 hours
Take with meals or just after to decrease gastric symptoms
Take early in the day to prevent nocturia and sleeplessness
Rx; Preg Cat B

Diabetic Medications

INSULIN

INSULIN, ZINC SUSPENSION EXTENDED (ULTRALENTE)

(Humulin U Ultralente, Novolin U, Ultralente U)

POTASSIUM-SPARING/COMBINATION DIURETICS

SPIRONOLACTONE

(speer-in-oh-lak-tone)

(Aldactone)

Side Effects

Hypoglycemia
Lipodystrophy

Nursing Considerations

Management of diabetes in patients allergic to other types of insulin and those disposed to thrombotic phenomena in which protamine may be a factor
Comes in 100 units per milliliter vial
subQ: Onset 1–2 1/2 hours, peak 7–15 hours, duration 18–24 hours
Not a replacement for regular insulin and is not suitable for emergency use
Rx; Preg Cat B

Side Effects

- Hyperkalemia
- Hyponatremia
- Vomiting, diarrhea
- Bleeding
- Rash, pruritus

Nursing Considerations

- Used in treatment of edema and hypertension
- Diuresis onset 24–48 hours, peak 48–72 hours
- Take in morning to avoid interference with sleep
- Take with meals or just after to decrease gastric symptoms
- Avoid food high in potassium: oranges, bananas, salt substitutes, dried apricots, dates
- Weigh daily to determine fluid loss; effect of drug may be decreased if used daily
- Contact clinician if cramps, lethargy, menstrual abnormalities, deepening voice, breast enlargement
- Rx; Preg Cat D

Diabetic Medications

INSULIN

INSULIN, ZINC SUSPENSION (LENTE)

(Humulin L, Novolin L)

POTASSIUM-SPARING/COMBINATION DIURETICS

TRIAMTERENE

(trye-am-ter-een)

(Dyrenium)

Side Effects

Hypoglycemia
Lipodystrophy

Nursing Considerations

Management of insulin-resistant diabetes requiring more than 200 units insulin per day
Comes in 500 units per milliliter vial
subQ: onset 1/2–1 hour, peak 2–5 hours, duration 5–7 hours
Deep secondary hypoglycemia 18–24 hours after injection; monitor closely and have 10–20% dextrose solution available
Record blood sugar 2 hour post-prandial
Rx; Preg Cat B

Side Effects

Nausea, vomiting, diarrhea
Anemia
Hyperkalemia

Nursing Considerations

Used in treatment of edema and hypertension
Diuresis onset 2 hours, peak 6–8 hours, duration 12–16 hours
Take with food if nausea develops, slight decrease in absorption
Take in morning to avoid interference with sleep
Avoid food high in potassium: oranges, bananas, salt substitutes, dried apricots, dates
Avoid prolonged exposure to sunlight; photosensitivity may occur, may turn urine blue
Weigh daily to determine fluid loss; effect of drug may be decreased if used daily
Rx; Preg Cat B

Diabetic Medications

INSULIN

INSULIN, REGULAR CONCENTRATED

(Iletin II U-500)

THIAZIDES/RELATED DIURETICS

CHLORTHALIDONE

(klor-thal-i-done)

(Hygroton, Hylidone, Thalitone; Tenoretic is combination with ATENOLOL)

Side Effects

Hypoglycemia
Lipodystrophy

Nursing Considerations

Management of diabetic coma, diabetic acidosis, or other emergency conditions. Esp. suitable for labile diabetes. Used in external insulin infusion pumps
Comes in 100 units per milliliter vial
Only insulin that can be given IV
subQ: onset 1/2–1 hour, peak 10–30 minutes, duration 1/2–1 hour
IV: onset 10–30 minutes, peak 10–30 minutes, duration 1/2–1 hour
Rx; Preg Cat B

Side Effects

Dizziness
Aplastic anemia
Orthostatic hypotension
Urinary frequency
Fatigue, weakness
Nausea, vomiting, anorexia
Electrolyte changes

Nursing Considerations

Used in treatment of edema and hypertension
Diuresis onset 2 hours, peak 6 hours, duration 24–72 hours
Take with meals or just after to decrease gastric symptoms
Blood sugar may increase in diabetics
Take in morning to avoid interference with sleep
Weigh daily to determine fluid loss; effect of drug may be decreased if used daily
Avoid changing positions (sitting/standing/lying) rapidly
Rx; Preg Cat B

Diabetic Medications

INSULIN

INSULIN, REGULAR

(Novolin R)

THIAZIDES/RELATED DIURETICS

HYDROCHLOROTHIAZIDE

(hye-droe-klor-oh-thye-a-zide)

(Hydrodiuril)

Side Effects

Hypoglycemia
Lipodystrophy

Nursing Considerations

Management of type 1 diabetes and in combination with sulfonylureas for type 2 diabetes
Take within 15 minutes of eating and immediately after mixing, with combined therapy
May be used in children in combination with sulfonylureas
Onset rapid, peak 1/2–1 1/2 hour, duration 6–8 hours
Rx; Preg Cat B

Side Effects

- Hypokalemia
- Hyperglycemia
- Blurred vision
- Fatigue, weakness
- Confusion, esp. in elderly
- Nausea, vomiting, anorexia

Nursing Considerations

- Used in treatment of edema and hypertension
- Diuresis onset 2 hours, peak 4 hours, duration 6–12 hours
- Take with meals or just after to decrease gastric symptoms
- Blood sugar may increase in diabetics
- Take in morning to avoid interference with sleep
- Use sunscreen to prevent photosensitivity
- Monitor for signs of hypokalemia: postural hypotension, malaise, fatigue, tachycardia, leg cramps, weakness, dehydration
- Rx; Preg Cat B

Diabetic Medications

INSULIN

INSULIN LISPRO

(Humalog)

THIAZIDES/RELATED DIURETICS

INDAPAMIDE

(in-dap-a-mide)

(Lozol)

Side Effects

Hypoglycemia
Lipodystrophy

Nursing Considerations

Management of diabetes
Comes in 100 units per milliliter vial as well as in combination with regular insulin in a 50/50 proportion and a 70/30 proportion
subQ: onset 1–1 1/2 hours, peak 4–12 hours, duration 18–24 hours
Rx; Preg Cat B

Side Effects

Headache
Electrolyte changes
Nausea
Rash, pruritus
Orthostatic hypotension

Nursing Considerations

Used in treatment of edema of CHF and hypertension
Diuresis onset 1–2 hours, peak 2 hours, duration 36 hours
Take with meals or just after to decrease gastric symptoms, slightly decreased absorption
Avoid changing positions (sitting/standing/lying) rapidly
Take in morning to avoid interference with sleep
Monitor for signs of hypokalemia: postural hypotension, malaise, fatigue, tachycardia, leg cramps, weakness, dehydration

Diabetic Medications

INSULIN

INSULIN, ISOPHANE SUSPENSION (NPH)

(Humulin N, Novolin N)

THIAZIDES/RELATED DIURETICS

METOLAZONE

(me-tole-a-zone)

(Diulo, Mykrox—prompt products, Zaroxolyn—extended product)

Side Effects

Hypoglycemia
Lipodystrophy

Nursing Considerations

Management of diabetes in type 1 diabetics or adults with type 2 requiring a long-acting insulin to control hyperglycemia
Onset 1.1 hours, peak 5 hours, duration 24 hours
Not the drug of choice for diabetic ketoacidosis (use a short-acting insulin)
Higher incidence of injection site pain compared with NPH
Rx; Preg Cat C

Side Effects

- Dizziness, weakness, fatigue
- Nausea, vomiting, anorexia
- Rash
- Hyperglycemia
- Hypokalemia

Nursing Considerations

- Used in treatment of edema of CHF and hypertension
- Diuresis onset 1 hour, peak 2 hours, duration 12–24 hours
- Take with meals or just after to decrease gastric symptoms, slightly decreased absorption
- Avoid changing positions (sitting/standing/lying) rapidly
- Take in morning to avoid interference with sleep
- Use sunscreen to prevent photosensitivity
- Monitor for signs of hypokalemia: postural hypotension, malaise, fatigue, tachycardia, leg cramps, weakness, dehydration
- Rx; Preg Cat B

Diabetic Medications

INSULIN

INSULIN GLARGINE

(Lantus)

Dermatologicals

ANTIFUNGALS, TOPICAL

KETOCONAZOLE

(key-toe-koe-na-zol)

(Nizoral)

Side Effects

Hypoglycemia

Lipodystrophy

Nursing Considerations

Management of diabetes in adults. The only insulin analog approved for use in external pump systems for continuous subQ insulin infusion.

Onset 15 minutes, peak 1–3 hours, duration 3–5 hours

Never administer IV

Immediately follow injection with meal within 5 to 10 minutes

Rx; Preg Cat B

Side Effects

Dizziness
Photophobia

Nursing Considerations

Treatment of fungal infections
C & S before first dose
PO: taken early A.M. with food
Also available as a topical cream or shampoo
Cannot take within two hours of alkaline substances, requires acid media to dissolve, follow with glass of water
Take at the same time each day
To prevent photophobia in bright sunlight, wear sunglasses
May require several weeks/months of therapy
Avoid use of alcohol
Rx; Preg Cat C

Diabetic Medications

INSULIN

INSULIN ASPART

(Novolog)

ANTIFUNGALS, TOPICAL

NYSTATIN

(nye-stat-in)

(Mycostatin)

Side Effects

Headache
Weakness, dizziness, drowsiness
Agitation
Nausea, vomiting, diarrhea
Lactic acidosis

Nursing Considerations

Management of stable adult-onset diabetes
PO: twice a day with meals to decrease GI upset and provide best absorption; may also be taken as one dose
Can crush tablets and mix with juice or soft foods for ease of swallowing
Do not crush, chew, or break extended release tablet; its coating may appear in stool
Be aware of signs of lactic acidosis: hyperventilation, fatigue, malaise, chills, myalgia, sleepiness
Have a quick source of sugar or a glucagon emergency kit available
Wear medical identification tag
Rx; Preg Cat B

Side Effects

GI distress, hypersensitivity

Nursing Considerations

Treatment of Candida infections
Discontinue if redness, swelling, irritation occurs
Encourage good oral, vaginal, skin hygiene
Rx; Preg Cat C

Diabetic Medications

HYPOGLYCEMIC AGENTS, ORAL

METFORMIN HCL

(met-for-min)

(Glucophage)

Dermatologicals

ANTI-INFLAMMATORIES, TOPICAL

FLUCINONIDE

(floo-oh-sin-oh-lone)

(Lidex)

Side Effects

Headache

Weakness, dizziness

Nursing Considerations

Management of stable adult-onset diabetes

Assess for symptoms of cholestatic jaundice: dark urine, pruritus, yellow sclera (rare)

Take at breakfast; onset is in 2 to 4 hours, peak in 4 hours, duration 24 hours

Have a quick source of sugar or a glucagon emergency kit available

Use sunscreen or protective clothing to prevent photosensitivity

Wear medical identification tag

Rx: Preg Cat B

Side Effects

Acne
Atrophy
Epidermal thinning
Purpura
Striae

Nursing Considerations

Topical glucorticoid used to treat severe dermatoses not responding to less potent meds: psoriasis, eczema, contact dermatitis, pruritus
Apply only to affected areas; do not get in eyes
Leave site uncovered or lightly covered
Occlusive dressing is not recommended, systemic absorption may occur
Do not use on weeping, denuded, or infected areas
Avoid sunlight on affected area
Rx; Preg Cat C

Diabetic Medications

HYPOGLYCEMIC AGENTS, ORAL

GLYBURIDE

(glye-byoo-ride)

(DiaBeta, Micronase)

TRIAMCINOLONE ACETONIDE

(trye-am-sin-oh-lone)

(Aristacort, Kenalog)

Side Effects

Headache

Weakness, dizziness

Drowsiness

Nursing Considerations

Management of stable adult-onset diabetes

Do not drink alcohol since it can produce a disulfiram reaction: nausea, headache, cramps, flushing, hypoglycemia

Assess for symptoms of cholestatic jaundice: dark urine, pruritus, yellow sclera (rare)

XL: take at breakfast; onset is in 1 to 1 1/2 hours, peak in 1 to 3 hours, duration 10–24 hours

Immediate release: take 30 minutes before meals, since absorption is delayed by food

Have a quick source of sugar or a glucagon emergency kit available

Use sun screen or protective clothing to prevent photosensitivity

Extended release tablet coating may appear in stool

Wear medical identification tag

Rx: Preg Cat C

Side Effects

- Acne
- Atrophy
- Epidermal thinning
- Purpura
- Striae

Nursing Considerations

- Topical glucorticoid used to treat severe dermatoses not responding to less potent meds: psoriasis, eczema, contact dermatitis, pruritus
- Apply only to affected areas; do not get in eyes
- Leave site uncovered or lightly covered
- Occlusive dressing is not recommended, systemic absorption may occur
- Do not use on weeping, denuded, or infected areas
- Avoid sunlight on affected area
- Rx; Preg Cat C

Diabetic Medications

HYPOGLYCEMIC AGENTS, ORAL

GLIPIZIDE

(glip-i-zide)

(Glucotrol)

HYPOGLYCEMIC AGENTS, ORAL

ACARBOSE

(ay-car-bose)

(Precose)

Side Effects

Headache

Weakness, dizziness

Drowsiness

Nursing Considerations

Management of stable adult-onset diabetes

Do not drink alcohol since it may produce a disulfiram reaction: nausea, headache, cramps, flushing, hypoglycemia

Assess for symptoms of cholestatic jaundice: dark urine, pruritus, yellow sclera (rare)

Take at breakfast or first main meal; onset is in 1 to 1 1/2 hours, peak in 1 to 3 hours, duration 10–24 hours

Have a quick source of sugar or a glucagon emergency kit available

Use sunscreen or protective clothing to prevent photosensitivity

Do not crush, chew or break extended release tablet; its coating may appear in stool

Wear medical identification tag

Rx: Preg Cat C

Side Effects

Abdominal pain
Diarrhea
Flatulence

Nursing Considerations

Management of diabetes by non-insulin dependent diabetics
Used alone or in combination with a sulfonylurea or insulin
PO: Take with first bite of each meal, med blood level peaks in 1 hour
Recognize signs of hypoglycemia: weakness, hunger, dizziness, tremors, anxiety, tachycardia, hunger, sweating
Treat hypoglycemia with dextrose, or if severe, IV glucose or glucagon
Measure short-term effectiveness with blood sugar one hour after meals
Measure long-term effectiveness with glycosylated Hgb every 3 months for the first year
Wear medical information tag
Rx, Preg Cat B

Diabetic Medications

HYPOGLYCEMIC AGENTS, ORAL

GLIMEPIRIDE

(glye-me-pi-ride)

(Amaryl)

APPENDIX A: LIST OF "DO NOT USE" ABBREVIATIONS FROM THE JOINT COMMISSION ON ACCREDITATION OF HEALTHCARE ORGANIZATIONS

One hundred percent compliance, in all forms of clinical documentation, with a reasonably comprehensive list of prohibited "dangerous" abbreviations, acronyms and symbols continues to be the long-term objective of the Joint Commission. Since January 1, 2005, the following items must be included on each accredited organization's "Do not use" list:

Abbreviation	Potential Problem	Preferred Term
U (for unit)	Mistaken as zero, four or cc.	Write "unit."
IU (for international unit)	Mistaken as IV (intravenous) or 10 (ten).	Write "international unit."
Q.D., Q.O.D. (Latin abbreviation for once daily and every other day)	Mistaken for each other. The period after the Q can be mistaken for an "I" and the "O" can be mistaken for "I."	Write "daily" and "every other day."
Trailing zero (X.0 mg), Lack of leading zero (.X mg)	Decimal point is missed.	Never write a zero by itself after a decimal point (X mg), and always use a zero before a decimal point (0.X mg).
MS	Can mean morphine sulfate or magnesium sulfate.	Write "morphine sulfate" or "magnesium sulfate."
MSO4 and MgSO4	Confused for one another.	Write "morphine sulfate" or "magnesium sulfate."

In addition to the “minimum required list,” the following items should also be considered for organizational “do not use” lists:

Abbreviation	Potential Problem	Preferred Term
> (greater than) < (less than)	Misinterpreted as the number “7” (seven) or the letter “L.” Confused for one another.	Write “greater than.” Write “less than.”
Abbreviations for drug names	Misinterpretated due to similiar abbreviations for multiple drugs.	Write drug names in full.
Apothecary units	Unfamiliar to many practitioners. Confused with metric units.	Use metric units.
@	Mistaken for the number “2” (two).	Write “at.”
cc	Mistaken for U (units) when poorly written.	Write “ml” for milliliters.
µg	Mistaken for mg (milligrams) resulting in one thousand-fold overdose.	“Write: “mcg” or “micrograms”

Note. An abbreviation on the "do not use" list should not be used in any of its forms—upper or lower case; with or without periods.

The Institute for Safe Medication Practices (ISMP) has published a list of dangerous abbreviations relating to medication use that it recommends should be explicitly prohibited. This list is available on the ISMP website: www.ismp.org.

APPENDIX B: CONTROLLED SUBSTANCE SCHEDULES

Drugs regulated by the Controlled Substances Act of 1970 are classified:

Schedule I: High abuse potential and no accepted medical use. Examples include heroin, marijuana, and LSD.

Schedule II: High abuse potential with severe dependence liability. Examples include narcotics, amphetamines, and some barbiturates.

Schedule III: Less abuse potential than schedule II drugs and moderate dependence liability. Examples include nonbarbiturate sedatives, nonamphetamine stimulants, anabolic steroids, and limited amounts of certain narcotics.

Schedule IV: Less abuse potential than schedule III drugs and limited dependence liability. Examples include some sedatives, anxiolytics, and nonnarcotic analgesics.

Schedule V: Limited abuse potential. Examples include small amounts of narcotics, such as codeine, used as antidiarrheals or antitussives.

APPENDIX C: PREGNANCY RISK CATEGORIES

The FDA has assigned the following pregnancy risk categories:

Category A: Adequate studies in pregnant women have failed to show a risk to the fetus in the first trimester (and there is not evidence of risk in later trimesters) and the possibility of fetal harm appears remote.

Category B: Animal studies haven't shown a risk to the fetus, but controlled studies haven't been conducted in pregnant women; or animal studies have shown an adverse effect on the fetus, but adequate studies in pregnant women haven't shown a risk to the fetus.

Category C: Animal studies have shown an adverse effect on the fetus, but adequate studies haven't been conducted in pregnant women. The benefits may be acceptable despite the risks.

Category D: The drug may cause a risk to the fetus, but potential benefits may be acceptable despite the risks (life-threatening situation or serious disease).

Category X: Animal or human studies show fetal abnormalities, or adverse reaction reports indicate evidence of fetal risk. The risks involved clearly outweigh potential benefits.

NA: Rating is not available

APPENDIX D: COMMON MEDICAL ABBREVIATIONS

ABC—airway, breathing, circulation

abd.—abdomen

ABG—arterial blood gas

ABO—system of classifying blood groups

ac—before meals

ACE—angiotensin converting enzyme

ACS—acute compartment syndrome

ACTH—adrenocorticotrophic hormone

ADH—antidiuretic hormone

ADL—activities of daily living

ad lib—freely, as desired

AFP—alpha-fetoprotein

AIDS—acquired immunodeficiency syndrome

AKA—above the knee amputation

ALL—acute lymphocytic leukemia

ALS—amyotrophic lateral sclerosis

ALT—alkaline phosphatase (formerly SGPT)

AMI—antibody-mediated immunity

AML—acute myelogenous leukemia

amt.—amount

ANA—antinuclear antibody

ANS—autonomic nervous system

AP—anteroposterior

A&P—anterior and posterior

APC—atrial premature contraction

aq.—water

ARDS—adult respiratory distress syndrome

ASD—atrial septal defect

ASHD—atherosclerotic heart disease

AST—aspartate aminotransferase (formerly SGOT)

ATP—adenosine triphosphate

AV—atrioventricular

BCG—Bacille Calmette-Guerin

bid—two times a day

BKA—below the knee amputation

BLS—basic life support

BMR—basal metabolic rate

BP—blood pressure

BPH—benign prostatic hypertrophy

bpm—beats per minute

BPR—bathroom privileges

BSA—body surface area

BUN—blood, urea, nitrogen

C—centigrade, Celsius

$\bar{c}$—with

Ca—calcium

CA—cancer

CABG—coronary artery bypass graft

CAD—coronary artery disease

CAPD—continuous ambulatory peritoneal dialysis

caps—capsules

CBC—complete blood count

CC—chief complaint

CCU—coronary care unit, critical care unit

CDC—Centers for Disease Control and Prevention

CHF—congestive heart failure

CK—creatine kinase

Cl—chloride

CLL—chronic lymphocytic leukemia

cm—centimeter

CMV—cytomegalovirus infection

CNS—central nervous system

CO—carbon monoxide, cardiac output

CO_2—carbon dioxide

comp—compound

cont—continuous

COPD—chronic obstructive pulmonary disease

CP—cerebral palsy

CPAP—continuous positive airway pressure

CPK—creatine phosphokinase

CPR—cardiopulmonary resuscitation

CRP—C-reactive protein

C&S—culture and sensitivity

CSF—cerebrospinal fluid

CT—computerized tomography

CTD—connective tissue disease

CTS—carpal tunnel syndrome

cu—cubic

CVA—cerebrovascular accident or costovertebral angle

CVC—central venous catheter

CVP—central venous pressure

DC—discontinue

D&C—dilation and curettage

DIC—disseminated intravascular coagulation

DIFF—differential blood count

dil.—dilute

DJD—degenerative joint disease

DKA—diabetic ketoacidosis

dL—deciliter (100 ml)

DM—diabetes mellitus

DNA—deoxyribonucleic acid

DNR—do not resuscitate

DO—doctor of osteopathy

DOE—dyspnea on exertion

DPT—vaccine for diphtheria, pertussis, tetanus

Dr.—doctor

DVT—deep vein thrombosis

D/W—dextrose in water

Dx—diagnosis

ECF—extracellular fluid

ECG or EKG—electrocardiogram

ECT—electroconvulsive therapy

ED—emergency department

EEG—electroencephalogram

EMD—electromechanical dissociation

EMG—electromyography

ENT—ear, nose, and throat

ESR—erythrocyte sedimentation rate

ESRD—end stage renal disease

ET—endotracheal tube

F—Fahrenheit

FBD—fibrocystic breast disease

FBS—fasting blood sugar

FDA—Food and Drug Administration

FFP—fresh frozen plasma

fl—fluid

4 × 4—piece of gauze 4" by 4" used for dressings

FSH—follicle-stimulating hormone

ft.—foot, feet (unit of measure)

FUO—fever of undetermined origin

g, gm—gram

GB—gall bladder

GFR—glomerular filtration rate

GH—growth hormone

GI—gastrointestinal

gr—grain

GSC—Glasgow coma scale

gtts—drops

GU—genitourinary

GYN—gynecological

h or hrs—hour or hours

(H)—hypodermically

Hb or Hgb—hemoglobin

HCG—human chorionic gonadotropin

HCO_3^-—bicarbonate

Hct—hematocrit

HD—hemodialysis

HDL—high-density lipoproteins

Hg—mercury

Hgb—hemoglobin

HGH—human growth hormone

HHNC—hyperglycemia hyperosmolar nonketotic coma

HIV—human immunodeficiency virus

HLA—human leukocyte antigen

HR—heart rate

hr—hour

HSV—herpes simplex virus

HTN—hypertension

H_2O—water

Hx—history

Hz—hertz (cycles/second)

IAPB—intra-aortic balloon pump

IBBP—intermittent positive pressure breathing

IBS—irritable bowel syndrome

ICF—intracellular fluid

ICP—increased intracranial pressure

ICS—intercostal space

ICU—intensive care unit

IDDM—insulin dependent diabetes mellitus

IgA—immunoglobulin A

IM—intramuscular

I&O—intake and output

IOP—increased intraocular pressure

IPG—impedance plethysmogram

IPPB—intermittent positive-pressure breathing

IUD—intrauterine device

IV—intravenous

IVC—intraventricular catheter

IVP—intravenous pyelogram

JRA—juvenile rheumatoid arthritis

K^+—potassium

kcal—kilocalorie (food calorie)

kg—kilogram

KO, KVO—keep vein open

KS—Kaposi's sarcoma

KUB—kidneys, ureters, bladder

L, l—liter

lab—laboratory

lb.—pound

LBBB—left bundle branch block

LDH—lactate dehydrogenase

LDL—low-density lipoproteins

LE—lupus erythematosus

LH—luteinizing hormone

liq—liquid

LLQ—left lower quadrant

LOC—level of consciousness

LP—lumbar puncture

LPN, LVN—licensed practical or vocational nurse

Lt, lt—left

LTC—long term care

LUQ—left upper quadrant

LV—left ventricle

m—minum, meter, micron

MAO—monoamine oxidase inhibitors

MAST—military antishock trousers

mcg—microgram

MCH—mean corpuscular hemoglobin

MCV—mean corpuscular volume

MD—muscular dystrophy, medical doctor

MDI—metered dose inhaler

mEq—milliequivalent

mg—milligram

Mg—magnesium

MG—myasthenia gravis

MI—myocardial infarction

ml—milliliter

mm—millimeter

MMR—vaccine for measles, mumps, rubella

MRI—magnetic resonance imaging

MS—multiple sclerosis

N—nitrogen, normal (strength of solution)

NIDDM—non-insulin dependent diabetes mellitus

Na^+—sodium

NaCl—sodium chloride

NANDA—North American Nursing Diagnosis Association

NG—nasogastric

NGT—nasogastric tube

NLN—National League for Nursing

noc—at night

NPO—nothing by mouth

NS—normal saline

NSAIDS—nonsteroidal anti-inflammatory drugs

NSNA—National Student Nurses' Association

NST—non-stress test

O_2—oxygen

OB-GYN—obstetrics and gynecology

OCT—oxytocin challenge test

OOB—out of bed

OPC—outpatient clinic

OR—operating room

$\overline{\text{os}}$—by mouth

OSHA—Occupational Safety and Health Administration

OTC—over the counter (drug that can be obtained without a prescription)

oz.—ounce

$\bar{p}$—with

P—pulse, pressure, phosphorus

PA Chest—posterior-anterior chest x-ray

PAC—premature atrial complexes

$PaCO_2$—partial pressure of carbon dioxide in arterial blood

PaO_2—partial pressure of oxygen in arterial blood

PAD—peripheral artery disease

Pap—Papanicolaou smear

pc—after meals

PCA—patient controlled analgesia

PCO_2—partial pressure of carbon dioxide

PCP—Pneumocystis carinii pneumonia

PD—peritoneal dialysis

PE—pulmonary embolism

PEEP—positive end-expiratory pressure

PERRLA—pupils equal, round, react to light and accommodation

PET—postural emission tomography

PFT—pulmonary function tests

pH—hydrogen ion concentration

PID—pelvic inflammatory disease

PKD—polycystic disease

PKU—phenylketonuria

PMS—premenstrual syndrome

PND—paroxysmal nocturnal dyspnea

PO, po—by mouth

PO_2—partial pressure of oxygen

PPD—positive purified protein derivative (of tuberculin)

PPN—partial parenteral nutrition

PRN, prn—as needed, whenever necessary

pro time—prothrombin time

PSA—prostate-specific antigen

psi—pounds per square inch

PSP—phenol-sulfonphthalein

PT—physical therapy, prothrombin time

PTCA—percutaneous transluminal coronary angioplasty

PTH—parathyroid hormone

PTT—partial thromboplastin time

PUD—peptic ulcer disease

PVC—premature ventricular contraction

q—every

QA—quality assurance

qh—every hour

q 2 h—every two hours

q 4 h—every four hours

qid—four times a day

qs—quantity sufficient

R—rectal temperature, respirations, roentgen

RA—rheumatoid arthritis

RAI—radioactive iodine

RAIU—radioactive iodine uptake

RAS—reticular activating system

RBBB—right bundle branch block

RBC—red blood cell or count

RCA—right coronary artery

RDA—recommended dietary allowance

resp—respirations

RF—rheumatic fever, rheumatoid factor

Rh—antigen on blood cell indicated by + or –

RIND—reversible ischemic neurologic deficit

RLQ—right lower quadrant

RN—registered nurse

RNA—ribonucleic acid

R/O, r/o—rule out, to exclude

ROM—range of motion (of joint)

Rt, rt—right

RUQ—right upper quadrant

Rx—prescription

$\overline{s}$—without

S. or Sig.—(Signa) to write on label

SA—sinoatrial node

SaO_2—systemic arterial oxygen saturation (%)

sat sol—saturated solution

SBE—subacute bacterial endocarditis

SDA—same day admission

SDS—same day surgery

sed rate—sedimentation rate

SGOT—serum glutamic-oxaloacetic transaminase (see AST)

SGPT—serum glutamic-pyruvic transaminase (see ALT)

SI—International System of Units

SIADH—syndrome of inappropriate antidiuretic hormone

SIDS—sudden infant death syndrome

SL—sublingual

SLE—systemic lupus erythematosus

SOB—short of breath

sol—solution

SMBG—self-monitoring blood glucose

SMR—submucous resection

sp gr—specific gravity

spec.—specimen

$\overline{ss}$—one half

SS—soap suds

SSKI—saturated solution of potassium iodide

stat—immediately

STD—sexually transmitted disease

subcut—subcutaneous

sx—symptoms

Syr.—syrup

T—temperature, thoracic to be followed by the number designating specific thoracic vertebra

T&A—tonsillectomy and adenoidectomy

tabs—tablets

TB—tuberculosis

T&C—type and crossmatch

TED—antiembolitic stockings

temp—temperature

TENS—transcutaneous electrical nerve stimulation

TIA—transient ischemic attack

TIBC—total iron binding capacity

tid—three times a day

tinct, or tr.—tincture

TMJ—temporomandibular joint

t-pa, TPA—tissue plasminogen activator

TPN—total parenteral nutrition

TPR—temperature, pulse, respiration

TQM—total quality management

TSE—testicular self-examination

TSH—thyroid-stimulating hormone

tsp—teaspoon

TSS—toxic shock syndrome

TURP—transuretheral prostatectomy

UA—urinalysis

ung—ointment

URI—upper respiratory tract infection

UTI—urinary tract infection

VAD—venous access device

VDRL—Veneral Disease Research laboratory (test for syphilis)

VF, Vfib—ventricular fibrillation

VPC—ventricular premature complexes

VS, vs—vital signs

VSD—ventricular septal defect

VT—ventricular tachycardia

WBC —white blood cell or count

WHO—World Health Organization

wt—weight